T0205481

Endocrine Pathophysiology

Andrea Manni • Akuffo Quarde

Endocrine Pathophysiology

A Concise Guide to the Physical Exam

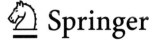

Springer

Andrea Manni
Division of Endocrinology
Diabetes and Metabolism
Penn State Milton S. Hershey
Medical Center
Hershey, PA
USA

Akuffo Quarde
Sanford Health Clinic
Bemidji, MN
USA

ISBN 978-3-030-49871-9   ISBN 978-3-030-49872-6   (eBook)
https://doi.org/10.1007/978-3-030-49872-6

This Springer imprint is published by the registered company Springer Nature Switzerland AG
The registered company address is: Gewerbestrasse 11, 6330 Cham, Switzerland

To my colleagues and trainees, who enriched my academic life.

To my wife, Rosemary, for her support throughout my career. – Andrea

To my beloved parents, for being inspiring forces in my life.

To my wife Anisa and children Stephanie and Nathan. – Akuffo

Preface

The physical exam is a dying art in modern medicine. In some instances, diagnostic tests and imaging procedures are significantly relied on at the expense of the physical examination. Hormone science (endocrinology) involves the study of perturbations in complex hormonal systems, which can present with a myriad of clinical signs. By bringing the pathophysiologic basis of clinical signs to the fore, we hope physicians in training can develop a better appreciation of the importance of the clinical exam.

Although modern medicine has improved our understanding of disease, the foundations laid by observant clinicians of a bygone era should be recognized by present-day clinicians. We have sought to highlight the contributions of various clinicians who have been pivotal in the development of this exciting field of clinical endocrinology.

We have strived to provide a concise approach to exploring endocrine pathophysiology through the physical exam and hope trainees and clinicians alike find the book an excellent addition to their library.

Hershey, PA, USA   Andrea Manni
Bemidji, MN, USA   Akuffo Quarde

Acknowledgments

We are grateful for the helpful suggestions and worthy contributions of various persons during the development of this book.

We appreciate the contributions of Dr. Alan Sacerdote (Retired Professor of Medicine, New York University School of Medicine), Dr. Chris Fan (Endocrinology Fellowship Director, Penn State University), Dr. Kanthi Bangalore Krishna (Assistant Professor of Medicine, Pediatric Endocrinology and Diabetes Division, Penn State University), Dr. Ariana Pichardo-Lowden (Associate Professor of Medicine, Endocrinology Division, Penn State University), and Dr. Shyam Narayana (Assistant Professor of Medicine, Endocrinology Division, Penn State University).

We sincerely appreciate the efforts of Dr. Avinindita Nura Lestari (Bachelor of Medicine, Universitas Islam Bandung, Indonesia) for designing and editing the illustrations. Her creative input and dedication to this project were commendable.

We want to thank Lisa Doster (Endocrinology Division, Penn State University) for her assistance during the writing of the manuscript.

We are also grateful to our publishing team at Springer and would like to say a special thank you to Kristopher Spring, Keerthana Gnanasekeran and Karthik Rajasekar.

Hershey, PA, USA   Andrea Manni
Bemidji, MN, USA   Akuffo Quarde

Contents

About the Authors

Andrea Manni MD – Professor of Medicine, Chief of the Division of Endocrinology, Diabetes and Metabolism, College of Medicine, The Pennsylvania State University, Hershey PA, USA. Email: amanni@pennstatehealth.psu.edu

Akuffo Quarde MD, PgD (Clinical Trials) – Endocrinologist, Sanford Health Clinic, Bemidji MN, USA. Email: akuffo.quarde@sanfordhealth.org

Pituitary Gland Signs

Learning Objectives

At the end of this chapter, you will be able to:

1. Understand the metabolic effects of growth hormone in both hormone excess and hormone-deficient states
2. Understand the role of growth hormone and other related hormones in the development of the growth plate
3. Identify the multiple effects of cortisol excess on the skin and integument
4. Recognize the concept of physiological cortisol resistance and its importance in specific endocrine conditions
5. Understand the effects of hyperprolactinemia on the hypothalamic-pituitary-gonadal axis
6. Recognize the pathophysiologic basis for the clinical presentation of central diabetes insipidus

1.1 Cushing's Disease

1.1.1 Proximal Myopathy

Clinical Features

Harvey Cushing reported muscle weakness as a cardinal finding in his original description of Cushing's disease [1, 2]. Proximal myopathy is an essential clinical clue in patients with overt hypercortisolism, with variable rates of prevalence ranging from 40 to 70% in retrospective studies [3, 4].

Proximal muscle weakness associated with Cushing's disease presents as an inability to either climb stairs or get up from a seated position without assistance. Loss of handgrip strength is also a known physical manifestation of Cushing's

© Springer Nature Switzerland AG 2020
A. Manni, A. Quarde, *Endocrine Pathophysiology*,
https://doi.org/10.1007/978-3-030-49872-6_1

disease, although pelvic girdle muscles are more likely to be involved than pectoral girdle and upper limb muscles [5, 6].

Pathophysiology
1. Glucocorticoids cause an increase in *muscle protein catabolism* resulting in a loss of lean body mass [7].
2. A reduction in *postabsorptive* and *post-prandial muscle protein synthesis* contributes to a loss of lean body mass as well [8].
3. Supraphysiologic levels of *glucocorticoids activate the mineralocorticoid receptor* at the level of the kidney, which results in hypokalemia (see Fig. 1.1). Hypokalemia-mediated muscle weakness contributes to the myopathy observed in endogenous hypercortisolism [9].
4. In Cushing's disease, aldosterone secretion is further augmented by adrenocorticotrophic hormone (ACTH) excess [10].

 Pathophysiology Pearl

Physiologic "Cortisol Resistance"
Cortisol can bind both glucocorticoid and mineralocorticoid receptors, and indeed under normal physiological conditions, plasma levels of cortisol are up to 1000-fold higher than that of aldosterone. 11Beta-hydroxysteroid dehydrogenase type 2 (11β-HSD2) inactivates physiological concentrations of cortisol and thus protects the mineralocorticoid receptor from direct activation by cortisol [11].

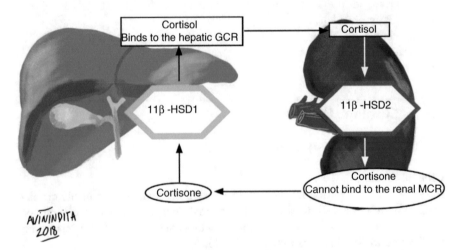

Fig. 1.1 The cortisol-to-cortisone shunt – the role of 11beta-hydroxysteroid dehydrogenases in mediating tissue-specific levels of cortisol. The two isoforms of 11beta-hydroxysteroid dehydrogenase play essential roles in the cortisol-to-cortisone shunt. 11Beta-hydroxysteroid dehydrogenase type 1 (11β HSD1) converts inactive cortisone to active cortisol in the liver, which subsequently binds its cognate hepatic glucocorticoid receptor (GCR)(dark arrows) [11]. 11Beta-hydroxysteroid dehydrogenase type 2 (11β HSD2) converts active cortisol to inactive cortisone at the level of the kidney, thus protecting the mineralocorticoid receptor (MCR) from activation by cortisol (white arrows) [12] (Redrawn and modified from Gomez-Sanchez et al. [11])

Table 1.1 Comparison of the isoforms of 11β HSD

11β HSD1	11β HSD2
Increases circulating levels of cortisol [15, 16]	Promotes physiological cortisol resistance [15]
Absent from the kidney [17]	Present in the kidney [17]
Absent from sweat and salivary glands [17]	Present in sweat and salivary glands [17]
Present in the liver [17]	Absent from the liver [17]
Present in osteoblasts and osteocytes [17]	Absent from the bone [17]
Present in adipose tissue [17]	Absent from adipose tissue [17]

11β HSD1 11beta-hydroxysteroid dehydrogenase type 1
11β HSD2 11beta-hydroxysteroid dehydrogenase type 2
Adapted from references [15–17]

In both ACTH-dependent and ACTH-independent Cushing's syndrome, there is an *impaired activity of 11β HSD2*, which leads to reduced deactivation of cortisol to cortisone in the kidney [9]. This defect results in a state of cortisol excess, akin to apparent mineralocorticoid excess (AME), or even licorice ingestion [13].

The excess cortisol thus stimulates the mineralocorticoid receptor. Increased mineralocorticoid action accounts for the hypokalemia observed in patients with hypercortisolemia [14] (Table 1.1).

 Clinical Pearl

Patients with adrenal crises because of Addison's disease do not require concomitant fludrocortisone (mineralocorticoid) administration if their total daily dose of steroids is greater than or equal to 50 mg of hydrocortisone, or *steroid equivalent*. Supraphysiologic doses of hydrocortisone, given during an emergency, will activate the mineralocorticoid receptor and thus provide additional *mineralocorticoid coverage*. Patients managed with *methylprednisolone* may and those taking *dexamethasone* will require mineralocorticoid due to limited binding of the former and zero binding of the latter to mineralocorticoid receptors [18].

1.1.2 Fat Maldistribution

Clinical Features
Visceral adiposity in the setting of endogenous hypercortisolism has been referred to as "Cushing's disease of the omentum" [19]. Abnormal fat distribution can also be disproportionately higher over the dorsocervical, supraclavicular, or temporal regions compared to the extremities [20].

Pathophysiology
1. Glucocorticoids inhibit a regulatory kinase involved in the sensing of cellular energy status. Under physiologic conditions, activation of adenosine 5'-monophosphate-activated protein kinase (AMPK) switches off fatty acid synthesis. Excess glucocorticoids inhibit AMPK and, by so doing, increase

fatty acid synthesis. This is a novel mechanism underlying the distribution of fat in Cushing's disease [21, 22].

2. There is overexpression of 11β HSD1 in visceral adipose tissue, which accounts for the excessive conversion of cortisone to cortisol in patients with Cushing's disease [23, 24] (see Fig. 1.1). Supraphysiologic levels of cortisol act in a paracrine fashion to increase fat storage in adipocytes, ultimately resulting in the accumulation of visceral fat [19]. The reasons for the preferential distribution of excess fat in the abdomen, head, and neck area, however, remain unclear.

1.1.3 Striae and Skin Atrophy

Clinical Features

Striae observed in Cushing's disease tend to be broad and violaceous, in contrast to the pale-colored thin striae associated with obesity. In darker-skinned individuals, striae may, however, not appear purple. Striae are typically distributed over the flanks, lower abdomen, upper thighs, and buttocks [25].

Skin atrophy can be assessed clinically by measuring skinfold thickness with a skin caliper [26]. Bedside assessment of skinfold thickness has been validated as an essential clinical tool in the evaluation of hypercortisolism. An improvised simple electrocardiographic caliper with its sharp edges blunted can be used to assess skinfold thickness over the proximal phalanx of the middle finger of the nondominant hand [27].

A skinfold thickness of 1.5 mm or lower is predictive of hypercortisolemia when comparing patients with Cushing's disease to controls without endogenous hypercortisolism [28].

In a recent paper, a skin thickness threshold of <2 mm was reported as being consistent with clinically significant thin skin. The positive likelihood ratio (+LR) for predicting endogenous hypercortisolism in patients with skin thickness less than 2 mm was estimated as 116 [27].

Pathophysiology

There are glucocorticoid receptors in the epidermis of the skin, located mainly on basal and Langerhans cells [29]. Activation of the glucocorticoid receptors present on these epidermal cells impairs collagen formation by reducing type 1 collagen gene expression; this leads to impaired skin growth and thinning of the epidermal layer [30].

1.1.4 Facial Plethora

Clinical Features

Facial plethora is a common clinical finding in patients with hypercortisolism [25] and is highly predictive of Cushing's disease. Of note, the other positive discriminatory findings of endogenous hypercortisolism include easy bruising, proximal myopathy, and purplish striae >1 cm [31].

Pathophysiology

Investigators at the National Institutes of Health (NIH) quantified vascular flow rates in patients with Cushing's syndrome, pre- and post-surgery. Patients with persistent facial plethora in the post-surgery period were noted to have cortisol levels above 3 mcg/dL, which was predictive of a lack of surgical cure. These subjects had a high facial blood volume fraction, measured by near-infrared multispectral imaging. Increased blood flow in the facial skin is the cause of plethora observed in the setting of endogenous hypercortisolism [32].

1.1.5 Hirsutism

Clinical Features

Hirsutism, a sign of androgen excess, is more common in the setting of adrenal carcinoma compared to Cushing's disease. Nonetheless, hirsutism in the right clinical context can be suggestive of endogenous hypercortisolemia [33]. Hirsutism presents in females as excessive terminal, pigmented hair growth, distributed in a classic male pattern [34].

Pathophysiology

ACTH-dependent Cushing's syndrome causes a mild form of hirsutism in women, through the trophic effect of corticotropin (ACTH) on the adrenal cortex. ACTH stimulates the zona reticularis resulting in increased biosynthesis of adrenal sex steroids [35] (Fig. 1.2).

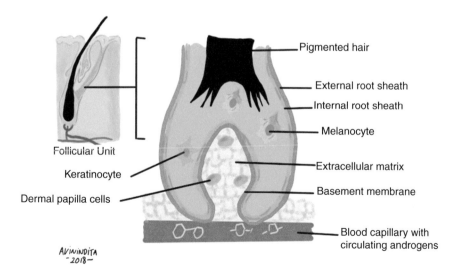

Fig. 1.2 Mechanism of androgen action in hair follicles. Circulating androgens access the dermal papilla cells via dermal capillaries. Androgens (testosterone or dihydrotestosterone) bind to specific target nuclear receptors in dermal papilla cells. Direct stimulation of keratinocytes and melanocytes occurs through androgen-mediated release of regulatory and growth-promoting factors from the dermal papilla cells [36]. (Based on Thornton et al. [36])

Associated Endocrinopathies/Differentials of Hirsutism
Congenital adrenal hyperplasia (CAH, both classical and nonclassical); polycystic ovarian syndrome (PCOS); Cushing's disease; acromegaly; insulin resistance; *hyperandrogenism, insulin resistance, and acanthosis nigricans* (HAIR-AN syndrome); and virilizing adrenal, ovarian, or ectopic tumors [34].

1.1.6 Hypertension

Clinical Features
80% of patients with Cushing's syndrome have hypertension. Of note, Cushing's-specific hypertension and primary hypertension may coexist in the same patient [37].

Pathophysiology
1. Supraphysiologic levels of cortisol overwhelm 11β-HSD2, an essential enzyme that protects the renal mineralocorticoid receptor from direct activation by glucocorticoids (see Fig. 1.1). Mineralocorticoid receptor activation eventually leads to excessive renal sodium and water conservation [14].
2. Glucocorticoids increase the plasma concentration of angiotensinogen and thus directly stimulate increased activity of the renin-angiotensin-aldosterone system (RAAS) [38].
3. Glucocorticoids increase the vasopressor effect of angiotensin II by stimulating messenger RNA expression of the angiotensin 1 (AT-1) receptor, the vascular receptor for angiotensin II [39].
4. Increased systemic vascular resistance due to glucocorticoid-mediated inhibition of vasodilatory pathways such as the nitric oxide system, kallikrein, and prostacyclin plays a contributory role as well [40].

1.1.7 Fragility Fractures

Clinical Features
Endogenous hypercortisolism increases the risk of low bone mineral density in a manner akin to exogenous glucocorticoid-induced osteoporosis (GIOP). Unlike exogenous GIOP, there is very little published literature on the prevalence of osteoporosis related-fractures in patients with Cushing's syndrome [41].

Pathophysiology
Endogenous hypercortisolism through various processes outlined below results in a low bone mineral density and predisposes patients to fragility fractures.

1. Decreased bone formation occurs because of increased glucocorticoid-mediated apoptosis of osteoblasts. There is also evidence that glucocorticoids directly inhibit the function of osteoblast as well [41].

2. Osteocytes which act as mechanoreceptors are also subject to apoptosis in the setting of high levels of glucocorticoids.
3. Glucocorticoids increase the expression of *receptor activator of nuclear factor κ-B ligand* (RANK-L) on the surface of osteoblasts with a concomitant reduction in osteoprotegerin (decoy-receptor for RANK-L) expression. The absence of the decoy receptor for RANK-L further potentiates osteoclastic activity, which ultimately promotes increased bone resorption and loss of bone mineral density (see Sect. 5.1.2) [41].

1.1.8   Hyperpigmentation

Clinical Features
Hyperpigmentation of the skin can occur in Cushing's disease, although it is more common in patients with ectopic ACTH production [42]. For patients with Cushing's disease, hyperpigmentation is common in those with persistent pituitary disease after bilateral adrenalectomy, i.e., Nelson's syndrome. Hyperpigmentation is usually evident in scars, buccal mucosa, conjunctivae, and sun-exposed areas [43, 44].

Pathophysiology
ACTH-induced hyperpigmentation has been described in detail (see Sect. 3.1.2).

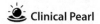 **Clinical Pearl**
Summary of the Clinical Features of Cushing's Disease (Fig. 1.3)

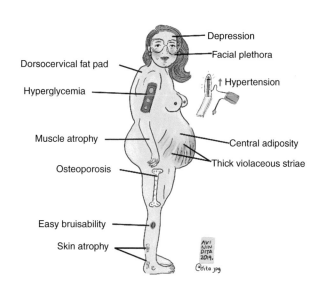

Fig. 1.3 Clinical features of Cushing's disease. The physical examination findings that are highly suggestive of Cushing's include proximal muscle weakness (myopathy), easy bruising, thick violaceous striae, and facial plethora [31]. (Based on Nieman et al. [31])

Questions You Might Be Asked on Clinical Rounds

Why would a patient with pituitary-dependent Cushing's develop adrenal insufficiency after adenomectomy?

A long duration of exposure of normal corticotrophs to supraphysiologic levels of cortisol results in suppression of their function through sustained negative feedback inhibition. Removal of the abnormal ACTH-producing cells contributes to loss of trophic stimulation of the zona fasciculata (cortisol producing layer of the adrenal gland). The remaining normal ACTH-producing cells are unable to sense low cortisol levels due to their chronic suppression by negative feedback inhibition; this explains the development of secondary adrenal insufficiency in patients during the postoperative period [45].

What is Nelson's syndrome?

Nelson's syndrome occurs after bilateral adrenalectomy to correct hypercortisolism in patients with Cushing's disease who have typically failed transsphenoidal surgery. It occurs as a result of the aggressive growth of the ACTH-producing adenoma following a loss of negative feedback inhibition by cortisol [46, 47].

Increased ACTH production and the mass effect of an expanding pituitary tumor contribute to the clinical features of this condition. These include hyperpigmentation, headaches, and visual field defects [48].

1.2   Acromegaly

1.2.1   Acanthosis Nigricans

Clinical Features
Patients with acromegaly exhibit some signs of insulin resistance. Acanthosis nigricans (AN) is a cardinal dermatologic feature of insulin resistance [49] and appears as a hyperpigmented, velvety skin lesion that has a predilection for flexural areas such as the neck, groin, and antecubital fossa [50, 51].

Pathophysiology
Growth hormone (GH) inhibits the phosphorylation of the insulin receptor in response to insulin-to-receptor binding, a process that contributes to the development of hyperinsulinemia [49].

The skin has several cells that express insulin-like growth factor 1 (IGF-1) receptors, including the stratum granulosum of the epidermis and dermal fibroblasts [52]. Excess insulin activates IGF-1 receptors in the skin and initiates the proliferation of dermal fibroblasts [53].

Associated Endocrinopathies/Differentials
Cushing's syndrome, acromegaly, PCOS, CAH, HAIR-AN syndrome, diabetes mellitus, paraneoplastic, and other hormonal causes of peripheral insulin resistance [51].

1.2.2 Frontal Bossing and Prognathism

Clinical Features
Frontal bossing and prognathism are cardinal craniofacial manifestations of acromegaly. Other signs include dental malocclusion and nasal bone hypertrophy [54]. In a study involving 29 acromegalics, the investigators assessed for any improvement in craniofacial skeletal deformities after curative tumor resection. Prespecified skull measurements did not differ significantly when the pre- and postsurgical dimensions were compared on serial magnetic resonance images (MRIs) [55]. These physical findings, unfortunately, will persist even after curative operative management of acromegaly, based on the results of this study.

Pathophysiology
Excess growth hormone and IGF-1 stimulate periosteal new bone formation resulting in the characteristic craniofacial features of acromegaly [54].

 Clinical Pearl
The Role of the "Photograph Biopsy"
    Acromegaly is a rare disease, which usually presents with a slow and progressive change in a patient's facial features. The diagnosis of acromegaly can be delayed by up to 10 years in most cases due to the subtle craniofacial changes seen in patients. In a recent study comparing over 500 acromegalic patients with an equivalent number of controls, the investigators used machine learning algorithms to predict the diagnosis of acromegaly in subjects with a high positive predictive value. Artificial intelligence software using facial recognition of serial photographs performed very well with both positive and negative predictive values well above 95% [56].

1.2.3 Acrochordons and Other Skin Manifestations

Clinical Features
Various cutaneous changes occur in acromegaly, including acrochordons (skin tags) and psoriasis [53]. Acrochordons, a sign of excessive soft tissue proliferation, may also point to the presence of synchronous colonic polyposis [54, 57]. Three or more skin tags in patients with a disease duration of 10 years are associated with a high pre-test probability for concomitant colonic polyposis [58]. Other skin and soft tissue manifestations include large lips or noses, oily skin, and hyperhidrosis (see Table 1.2) [59].

Table 1.2 Mechanisms underlying other manifestations of acromegaly

Physical sign	Mechanism
Skin thickening	Deposition of glycosaminoglycans in the skin [58]
Sweaty or oily skin	IGF-1-mediated hypertrophy of sebaceous and sweat glands [58]
Hirsutism	GH causes reduced production of sex hormone-binding globulin (SHBG), most likely because of GH-induced hyperinsulinemia. This leads to excess circulating free androgens due to the reduced fraction of SHBG (see Sect. 1.1.5) [68] Excess circulating IGF-1 causes insulin resistance and consequent hyperinsulinemia. Hyperinsulinemia potentiates the production of androgens from the ovaries [68]
Goiter	GH and IGF-1 have growth stimulatory effects on thyroid follicular cells [69]

Adapted from references [58, 68, 69]

Pathophysiology
1. The action of IGF-1 on skin cells causes an accumulation of dermal glycosaminoglycans, which accounts for the characteristic soft tissue changes noted on the face, hands, and feet [53].
2. The mechanism underlying skin tag formation is unclear. It may be due to IGF-1 acting on its receptors present on skin cells, which ultimately leads to a proliferation of dermal fibroblasts. An alternative explanation is growth hormone excess, contributing to an insulin-resistant state, which promotes hyperinsulinemia-mediated skin tag formation (see Sect. 4.1.3) [59, 60].

1.2.4   Colonic Polyps

Clinical Features
There is a reported excess risk of premalignant colonic adenomas in patients with acromegaly compared to the general population [61].

Pathophysiology
IGF-1, through its potentiation effects on colonic epithelial cell proliferation, increases the risk of colonic polyp formation [61].

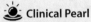 Clinical Pearl

The Endocrine Society recommends a **baseline colonoscopy screen at the time of diagnosis** and every 5 years if there is persistently elevated IGF-1 or the presence of a colonic polyp at the initial screening colonoscopy. In the absence of colonic polyps or persistent elevation of IGF-1, the recommendation is to screen every 10 years [62].

1.2.5 Tinel's Sign (Carpal Tunnel Syndrome)

Clinical Features
Nerve entrapment syndromes like carpal tunnel syndrome (CTS) and ulnar nerve neuropathy occur in acromegalics. CTS has a prevalence of 20 to 64% in patients with acromegaly [63]. Positive Tinel's sign is the presence of reproducible median nerve compressive symptoms (tingling sensation involving the first three and a half digits) upon tapping the location of the median nerve, just proximal to the wrist joint. Tinel's sign has positive and negative predictive values of 88% and 76%, respectively [64].

Pathophysiology
This compressive neuropathy based on clinical studies involving an imaging modality has been attributed to edema of the perineural sheath and not mere soft tissue proliferation in the wrist joint [63]. In a paper published in the *Annals of Internal Medicine*, researchers investigated the reason for CTS seen in acromegaly [65].

Magnetic resonance images (MRIs) of the wrists, at baseline, were compared to repeat images at 6 months post-treatment. The dimensions of soft tissue in the wrist were no different between acromegalics with and without CTS. There was, however, an improvement in perineural edema, making it the underlying cause of the neuropathic complaints, and not soft tissue swelling [65].

1.2.6 Hypertension

Clinical Features
Hypertension increases the risk of cardiovascular mortality in patients with acromegaly [66], with an estimated prevalence of 33–46% [62].

Pathophysiology
1. Increased plasma volume because of the activation of the renin-angiotensin-aldosterone axis by excess growth hormone [66].
2. Excess IGF-1 also promotes the growth of cardiomyocytes (cardiac remodeling) [66].
3. Insulin resistance in the setting of acromegaly contributes to vascular smooth muscle proliferation and vasculopathy [66].
4. Increased cardiac inotropy occurs because of IGF-1-mediated potentiation of calcium effects in the contractile units of the heart [66].
5. Obstructive sleep apnea due to soft tissue proliferation in the head and neck region contributes to hypertension [67].

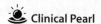 **Clinical Pearl**
Acromegaly is associated with other physical manifestations, including hyperhidrosis, hirsutism, goiter, and skin thickening.

Questions You Might Be Asked on Clinical Rounds

Approximately 30% of patients with acromegaly have hyperprolactinemia. What are the reasons for this [70]?

1. Co-secretion of growth hormone and prolactin by the tumor may occur in patients with acromegaly due to the common embryologic origin of mammosomatotroph cells.
2. Compression of the pituitary stalk by a macroadenoma impairs dopamine-mediated tonic inhibition of prolactin secretion (stalk effect) [70].

What are the familial syndromes associated with growth hormone hypersecretion [58]?
Carney complex, multiple endocrine neoplasia (MEN) type 1, McCune-Albright syndrome, and familial isolated acromegaly [58]

1.3   Prolactinoma

1.3.1   Hypogonadism

Clinical Features
Prolactinomas usually present with hypogonadal symptoms in men. These include erectile dysfunction, infertility, and decreased libido [71]. Premenopausal women may have either oligomenorrhea or amenorrhea [72].

Pathophysiology
1. Hyperprolactinemia reduces the pulse frequency and amplitude of luteinizing hormone (LH) and follicle-stimulating hormone (FSH) through its inhibitory action on gonadotrophin-releasing hormone (GnRH) neurons in the hypothalamus [73].
2. Prolactin directly inhibits the synthesis of gonadal steroids leading to hypogonadism [74]. Interestingly, prolactin stimulates adrenal androgen synthesis by potentiating the effect of ACTH on the zona reticularis, although this contributory effect of prolactin on steroidogenesis is not very significant [75].

1.3.2   Gynecomastia and Galactorrhea

Clinical Features
Galactorrhea is defined as the secretion of a milky fluid from the breast either spontaneously or with manual expression, in the absence of gestation [76]. Galactorrhea occurs in both men and women, although it tends to be more prevalent in the latter. Gynecomastia is the benign growth of male breast glandular tissue [31].

Pathophysiology
Prolactin binds to its receptors on mammary epithelial cells, which happen to be embryologic derivatives of keratinocytes. This stimulates glandular tissue proliferation resulting in gynecomastia (men) and galactorrhea (both men and women) [77, 78].

Galactorrhea is less common in men compared to women because of the lack of estrogen and progesterone primed glandular breast tissue in the former compared to the latter [77].

1.3.3 Bitemporal Hemianopsia

Clinical Features
Bitemporal hemianopsia presents as a loss of peripheral vision. The presence of this peripheral scotoma may impact a patient's functional status negatively, including the ability to drive a motor vehicle [79]. It is best measured by conventional perimetry [79], although a simple bedside visual field confrontation test can be helpful in the initial assessment [80].

The classic presentation of bitemporal hemianopsia is rare in patients with visual field defects due to a pituitary macroadenoma [81–83]. In a recent retrospective study comparing pituitary MRI findings with formal visual field records, the authors reported other visual field defects as being more likely even in the presence of significant optic chiasmal compression, defined as a chiasmal displacement greater than 3 mm. Interestingly, a single patient out of a cohort of 115 had the classic presentation of bitemporal hemianopsia, despite the evidence of chiasmal compression. These findings are indeed inconsistent with the long-held view of bitemporal hemianopsia being the likely visual field defect in the setting of chiasmal compression [84].

Pathophysiology
The classic presentation of bitemporal hemianopsia occurs because of the unique anatomic position of the optic chiasm with relation to the pituitary gland and the intricate neuronal innervation of both the temporal and nasal visual fields by the optic nerve [83].

 Questions You Might Be Asked on Clinical Rounds
What are the mechanisms underlying the increased risk of fragility fractures in patients with prolactinomas?
Hypogonadism is the cardinal reason for low bone mineral density in patients with prolactinomas. Also, prolactin impairs the proliferation of osteoblasts and may, in some instances, contribute to apoptosis of these cells [85].

How does hyperprolactinemia cause hirsutism?

- Prolactin receptors are present on dermal papilla cells and keratinocytes. Prolactin-to-prolactin receptor binding induces active hair growth through stimulation of dermal papilla cells, a process that results in the proliferation of keratinocytes [78].
- Prolactin directly induces adrenal androgen synthesis [75].

1.4 Adult Growth Hormone Deficiency

1.4.1 Abnormal Body Composition

Clinical Features
Adult growth hormone deficiency (AGHD) is characterized by increased visceral adiposity (abdominal obesity) and a low lean body mass [86, 87].

Pathophysiology
1. Growth hormone (GH) plays an essential role in lipolysis by modulating the activity of both lipoprotein and hormone-sensitive lipases. GH inhibits the activity of lipoprotein lipase (LPL) in adipose tissue (*GH deficiency promotes fat storage*). Also, the inhibitory role of insulin on hormone-sensitive lipase (HSL) activity is further enhanced by GH action (*GH deficiency inhibits fat mobilization*) [88, 89] (see Fig. 1.4). The exact mechanism underlying the excessive storage of fat in adipose tissue as occurs in AGHD, however, remains unclear. What is known is that patients with AGHD have a higher fat cell volume, but a relatively lower fat cell number, when compared to matched controls without growth hormone deficiency. In summary, growth hormone deficiency causes a net effect of increased lipid storage in adipose tissue [90].
2. GH increases protein synthesis; it, however, remains unclear if GH stimulates protein synthesis in all tissues. Impaired GH-mediated protein synthesis explains, in part, the loss of lean body mass in patients with AGHD [91].

☀ Clinical Pearl
Management of Hypertriglyceridemia-Induced Pancreatitis
   A continuous intravenous insulin infusion is used in treating significant hypertriglyceridemia-induced acute pancreatitis. Insulin augments the action of LPL, which facilitates the transfer of TAG-rich lipoproteins such as chylomicrons and VLDL from the circulation into fat stores in adipose tissue (see Fig. 1.4) [92].

Questions You Might Be Asked on Clinical Rounds

Does adult growth hormone deficiency lead to low bone mineral density [93]?

AGHD does not cause low bone mineral density. There is a paucity of randomized controlled trials (RCTs) investigating the effects of growth hormone replacement therapy on fragility fracture risk in AGHD [93].

Do quality of life (QoL) scores improve after growth hormone replacement therapy in patients with AGHD?

There is a variable response in QoL scores across a heterogeneous patient population with AGHD. Patients either develop worse scores, remain the same, or improve [93].

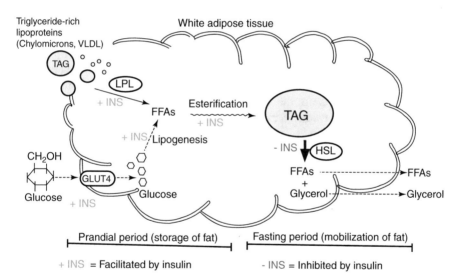

Fig. 1.4 Schematic diagram of the role of LPL and HSL in fat storage and mobilization. LPL is synthesized in adipocyte tissue and is then transported to its site of action, which is the luminal surface of the capillary endothelium. LPL is involved in the uptake of fatty acids into adipose tissue by mediating the hydrolysis of triacylglycerol (TAG) laden lipoproteins into free fatty acids (FFAs) (thin arrow). Glucose transporter 4 (GLUT4) mobilizes glucose from the peripheral circulation for lipogenesis in adipose tissue. This occurs in the fed state and is facilitated by insulin (dotted arrows). The esterification of FFAs into TAG is potentiated by insulin (wavy arrow). Hormone-sensitive lipase (HSL) mediates the conversion of TAG into glycerol and FFAs (thick arrow) for subsequent release into the bloodstream (dashed arrows). This process of fat mobilization occurs in the fasting state and is inhibited by insulin [89]. (Redrawn and modified from Frayn et al. [89])

1.5   Growth Hormone Insensitivity (Laron-Type Dwarfism)

1.5.1   Short Stature

Clinical Features
Laron-type dwarfism is the most severe form of growth hormone insensitivity and was first described in 1966. Children born with Laron dwarfism have a growth velocity of less than 50% of their predicted rate [94]. Patients are of short stature with a final height being −4 to −8 standard deviations below the normal for their age and gender [95].

Pathophysiology
Mutation of the growth hormone receptor (GHR) gene results in resistance to the systemic effects of growth hormone. Patients with GH insensitivity have high circulating levels of GH with very low IGF-1 levels [94, 96].

1. The role of growth hormone in stimulating chondrocytes in the proliferative zone of the growth plate is impaired in growth hormone insensitivity [97, 98].
2. Local IGF-1 production in the growth plate is impaired because of an absence of the stimulating effects of growth hormone in the setting of a mutation of the GHR [97]. Disruption of the stimulatory paracrine effects of IGF-1 on growth plate chondrocytes results in impaired linear growth [98, 99].

 Pathophysiology Pearl

Growth Plate Physiology and the Hormonal Milieu
   Growth hormone (GH) secretion from the anterior pituitary somatotrophs is under trophic stimulation by hypothalamic-derived growth hormone-releasing hormone (GHRH). GH binds to receptors in the liver, leading to hepatic production of IGF-1, which mediates the peripheral effects of GH. GH acts locally in the growth plate of the bone to stimulate local IGF-1 production, which, through its paracrine effects, plays a vital role in linear growth [97, 99] (Fig. 1.5).

1.5.2   Obesity

Clinical Features
Obesity in subjects with Laron dwarfism worsens progressively with age [96]. Patients have a higher proportion of body fat compared to age- and gender-matched healthy controls [103]. Dr. Zvi Laron and colleagues reported severe obesity as a cardinal clinical sign in both children and adults with Laron dwarfism [104].

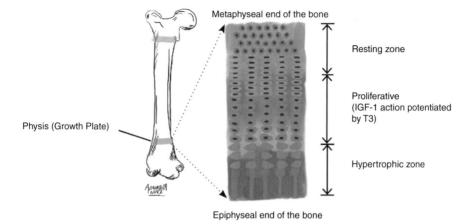

Fig. 1.5 Physiologic zones of the growth plate. The growth plate is composed of three zones, the resting, proliferative, and hypertrophic zones. Bone formation is a gradual process of differentiation and maturation of chondrocytes in the growth plate, with a progressive transition from the epiphyseal (articular end of the bone) to the metaphyseal end (main shaft of the bone) [100]. Progenitor cells in the resting zone are destined to become more matured chondrocytes in the proliferative zone under the influence of hormonal signals, including thyroid hormone, androgens, estrogens, GH, and IGF-1 [101].Chondrocytes in the hypertrophic zone are terminally differentiated and, in due time, undergo apoptosis. Eventually, chondrocytes are no longer able to lay down the matrix needed for new bone formation, leading to complete fusion of the epiphyses [102]. The role of thyroid hormone and estrogens has been described elsewhere (see Sects. 2.4.2 and 6.5.1, respectively). (Redrawn and modified from Long et al [100])

Pathophysiology
1. The reasons for the increased incidence of obesity in subjects with Laron dwarfism remains unclear [104]. However, since GH increases lean body mass and the muscle/fat ratio, it is plausible that a lack of GH effect would cause the opposite effect, i.e., a low muscle to fat ratio [105].
2. A study by Dr. Laron and his group discounted the reasons for obesity as being due to either hyperphagia or reduced metabolism. They also measured the resting energy expenditure in patients with growth hormone insensitivity and found it be unexpectedly higher than was predicted based on the lean body mass of subjects [103].

1.5.3   Small Genitalia

Clinical Features
There is a delayed but eventual achievement of full sexual maturity. The male testis reaches a final adult size of 5-9 ml, which is lower than that of healthy subjects [104]; nonetheless, both sexes can still achieve fertility in adulthood [104, 106].

Pathophysiology

Testicular growth and development are influenced by endocrine and paracrine effects of IGF-1, although the exact mechanisms are yet to be elucidated. There are indeed IGF-1 receptors present on Sertoli cells of the testis [107]. The importance of trophic stimulation of the Sertoli cells in determining the final testicular volume has been described in Sect. 6.3.1.

 Questions You Might Be Asked on Clinical Rounds

What is the reason for a low risk of cancers seen in patients with congenital growth hormone receptor deficiency (GHRD)?

In a prospective cohort study of 99 subjects with growth hormone receptor deficiency (Laron dwarfism) followed up for more than two decades, cancer-related deaths did not occur. The authors tested in vitro human mammary epithelial cells and were able to demonstrate that reduced IGF-1 signaling resulted in programmed cell death of epithelial cells whose DNA had been damaged by pretreatment with hydrogen peroxide. IGF-1 signaling prevents apoptosis of damaged DNA and therefore increases the risk of carcinogenesis [108]. Interestingly, clinical trials investigating the use of monoclonal antibodies directed against the IGF-1 signaling pathway have not been consistently successful in cancer therapy [109].

What is the reason for the low risk of diabetes mellitus seen in patients with congenital GHRD?

In another prospective cohort of patients with congenital growth receptor deficiency followed up for more than two decades, despite having disproportionately high body fat, subjects demonstrated increased insulin sensitivity. None of the subjects had diabetes mellitus. Interestingly, other measures of insulin resistance, such as the homeostatic model assessment of insulin resistance (HOMA-IR), triglycerides, and glucose levels, were all lower than age- and sex-matched controls. GHRD impairs the counterregulatory effects of GH on glucose metabolism; this may explain the absence of diabetes in these patients [110]. Might an anti-IGF-1 monoclonal antibody be a potential future diabetes therapy?

1.6   Central Diabetes Insipidus

1.6.1   Dehydration due to Polyuria and Polydipsia

Clinical Features

Patients with central diabetes insipidus present with hypotonic polyuria and polydipsia. Excessive free water loss leads to clinical signs suggestive of dehydration [111].

Pathophysiology

1. Downregulation of vasopressin V2 receptors in the principal cell of the collecting tubule occurs due to the absence of trophic stimulation by arginine vasopressin (AVP), in the setting of complete central diabetes insipidus. Also, a loss of AVP stimulation causes internalization of aquaporin-2 (AQP2) water channels into cytosolic vesicles, which ultimately leads to free water loss (see Fig. 1.6) [112, 113].

2. Additionally, AVP in high concentrations, as might occur during periods of shock, binds to V1 receptors in vascular smooth muscle. V1 receptor activation causes smooth muscle contraction and maintenance of blood pressure [115].

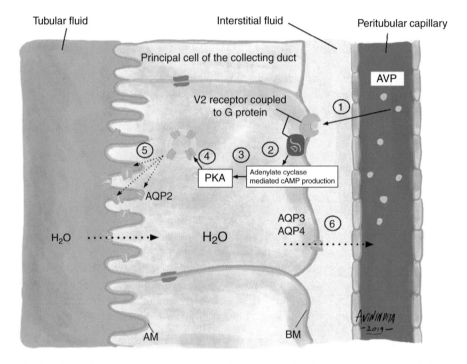

Fig. 1.6 The role AVP in renal water conservation at the renal collecting duct cell. AVP binds to the G-protein-coupled V2 receptor on the basolateral membrane of the principal cell (step 1). This is followed by the activation of cytosolic adenylate cyclase, which subsequently increases cyclic AMP (cAMP) production (step 2). Increased intracellular cAMP activates Protein Kinase A (PKA) (step 3), which then facilitates the phosphorylation of AQP2 in its endocytic vesicles (step 4). AQP2 liberated from endocytic vesicles are translocated to the apical membrane (AM) of the principal cell (step 5). AQP3 and AQP4 are constitutively expressed (not released from endocytic vesicles) on the basolateral membrane, independent of PKA action. AQP2 moves free water from the collecting tubule into the cytosol of the ductal cell, while AQP3 and AQP4 water channels mediate the movement of free water across the basolateral membrane into the peritubular capillaries (step 6) [114]. (Redrawn and modified from Moritz et al [114])

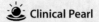 **Clinical Pearl**

The Triphasic Response of Central Diabetes Insipidus
Complete transection of the pituitary stalk, as might occur in traumatic brain injury or transsphenoidal surgery, results in the classic "triphasic response" of central diabetes insipidus.

- There is an initial phase of *transient central diabetes insipidus*, which occurs due to axonal shock.
- The first phase is followed within 24 to 48 hours by a second phase of *syndrome of inappropriate antidiuretic hormone (SIADH)*, due to axonal injury and rapid release of preformed AVP into circulation.
- The third phase of *recurrence of central diabetes insipidus* occurs after the complete depletion of neuronal reserves of AVP.

The challenge in managing this condition is realizing the clinical timeline of the triphasic response and altering fluid management promptly to prevent acute sodium imbalance [116].

 Questions You Might Be Asked on Clinical Rounds

With regard to desmopressin supplementation in the management of central diabetes insipidus, what precautions should be taken in patients on concomitant nonsteroidal anti-inflammatory drugs (NSAIDs)?
Patients should be informed of suitable alternatives to NSAIDs when on long-term stable doses of desmopressin therapy. Clinicians taking care of patients should also be aware of the risk of water intoxication and severe hyponatremia when patients on desmopressin receive NSAIDs [117].

How do prostaglandins impact water conservation in the kidney?
Prostaglandin E2 (PGE2) plays a critical role in inhibiting the effects of AVP in the collecting ducts. NSAIDs inhibit prostaglandin synthesis, which results in an exaggeration of AVP effects in the renal collecting system, a process that promotes water intoxication and hyponatremia [118].

It is worthy to note that up to 85% of glomerular filtrate reabsorption is *AVP-independent* and occurs in the proximal tubules and descending limbs of the loop of Henle. *AVP-dependent* mechanisms, although accounting for only 15% of water reabsorption at the level of the collecting ducts, contribute significantly to sodium balance [112, 119].

References

1. Müller R, Kugelberg E. Myopathy in Cushing's syndrome. J Neurol Neurosurg Psychiatry. 1959;22:314–9.
2. Cushing H. The basophil adenomas of the pituitary body. Ann R Coll Surg Engl. 1969;44:180–1.
3. Bolland MJ, Holdaway IM, Berkeley JE, Lim S, Dransfield WJ, Conaglen JV, Croxson MS, Gamble GD, Hunt PJ, Toomath RJ. Mortality and morbidity in Cushing's syndrome in New Zealand. Clin Endocrinol. 2011;75:436–42.
4. Ammini AC, Tandon N, Gupta N, et al. Etiology and clinical profile of patients with Cushing's syndrome: a single center experience. Indian J Endocrinol Metab. 2014;18:99.
5. Berr CM, Stieg MR, Deutschbein T, et al. Persistence of myopathy in Cushing's syndrome: evaluation of the German Cushing's registry. Eur J Endocrinol. 2017;176:737–46.
6. Minetto MA, Lanfranco F, Motta G, Allasia S, Arvat E, D'Antona G. Steroid myopathy: some unresolved issues. J Endocrinol Investig. 2011;34:370–5.
7. Fitts RH, Romatowski JG, Peters JR, Paddon-Jones D, Wolfe RR, Ferrando AA. The deleterious effects of bed rest on human skeletal muscle fibers are exacerbated by hypercortisolemia and ameliorated by dietary supplementation. Am J Physiol-Cell Physiol. 2007;293:C313–20.
8. Phillips SM, Glover EI, Rennie MJ. Alterations of protein turnover underlying disuse atrophy in human skeletal muscle. J Appl Physiol. 2009;107:645–54.
9. Stewart PM, Walker BR, Holder G, O'Halloran D, Shackleton CH. 11 beta-Hydroxysteroid dehydrogenase activity in Cushing's syndrome: explaining the mineralocorticoid excess state of the ectopic adrenocorticotropin syndrome. J Clin Endocrinol Metab. 1995;80:3617–20.
10. Sharma ST, Nieman LK. Cushing's syndrome: all variants, detection, and treatment. Endocrinol Metab Clin N Am. 2011;40:379–91.
11. Gomez-Sanchez E, Gomez-Sanchez CE. The multifaceted mineralocorticoid receptor. Compr Physiol. 2014;4:965–94.
12. Stewart PM, Murry BA, Mason JI. Human kidney 11 beta-hydroxysteroid dehydrogenase is a high affinity nicotinamide adenine dinucleotide-dependent enzyme and differs from the cloned type I isoform. J Clin Endocrinol Metab. 1994;79:480–4.
13. Stewart PM. Tissue-specific Cushing's syndrome, 11beta-hydroxysteroid dehydrogenases and the redefinition of corticosteroid hormone action. Eur J Endocrinol. 2003;149:163–8.
14. Frey FJ, Odermatt A, Frey BM. Glucocorticoid-mediated mineralocorticoid receptor activation and hypertension. Curr Opin Nephrol Hypertens. 2004;13:451–8.
15. Tomlinson JW, Stewart PM. Cortisol metabolism and the role of 11β-hydroxysteroid dehydrogenase. Best Pract Res Clin Endocrinol Metab. 2001;15:61–78.
16. Loerz C, Maser E. The cortisol-activating enzyme 11β-hydroxysteroid dehydrogenase type 1 in skeletal muscle in the pathogenesis of the metabolic syndrome. J Steroid Biochem Mol Biol. 2017;174:65–71.
17. Draper N, Stewart PM. 11beta-hydroxysteroid dehydrogenase and the pre-receptor regulation of corticosteroid hormone action. J Endocrinol. 2005;186:251–71.
18. Arlt W. The approach to the adult with newly diagnosed adrenal insufficiency. J Clin Endocrinol Metab. 2009;94:1059–67.
19. Bujalska IJ, Kumar S, Stewart PM. Does central obesity reflect "Cushing's disease of the omentum"? Lancet Lond Engl. 1997;349:1210–3.
20. Baid SK, Rubino D, Sinaii N, Ramsey S, Frank A, Nieman LK. Specificity of screening tests for Cushing's syndrome in an overweight and obese population. J Clin Endocrinol Metab. 2009;94:3857–64.
21. Kahn BB, Alquier T, Carling D, Hardie DG. AMP-activated protein kinase: ancient energy gauge provides clues to modern understanding of metabolism. Cell Metab. 2005;1:15–25.

22. Kola B, Christ-Crain M, Lolli F, Arnaldi G, Giacchetti G, Boscaro M, Grossman AB, Korbonits M. Changes in adenosine 5′-monophosphate-activated protein kinase as a mechanism of visceral obesity in Cushing's syndrome. J Clin Endocrinol Metab. 2008;93:4969–73.

23. Tomlinson JW, Draper N, Mackie J, Johnson AP, Holder G, Wood P, Stewart PM. Absence of Cushingoid phenotype in a patient with Cushing's disease due to defective cortisone to cortisol conversion. J Clin Endocrinol Metab. 2002;87:57–62.

24. Anagnostis P, Katsiki N, Adamidou F, Athyros VG, Karagiannis A, Kita M, Mikhailidis DP. 11beta-Hydroxysteroid dehydrogenase type 1 inhibitors: novel agents for the treatment of metabolic syndrome and obesity-related disorders? Metab - Clin Exp. 2013;62:21–33.

25. Thiboutot DM. Clinical review 74: dermatological manifestations of endocrine disorders. J Clin Endocrinol Metab. 1995;80:3082–7.

26. Dykes PJ, Marks R. Measurement of skin thickness: a comparison of two in vivo techniques with a conventional histometric method. J Invest Dermatol. 1977;69:275–8.

27. Loriaux DL. Diagnosis and differential diagnosis of Cushing's syndrome. N Engl J Med. 2017;376:1451–9.

28. Corenblum B, Kwan T, Gee S, Wong NCW. Bedside assessment of skin-fold thickness: a useful measurement for distinguishing Cushing's disease from other causes of hirsutism and Oligomenorrhea. Arch Intern Med. 1994;154:777–81.

29. Serres M, Viac J, Schmitt D. Glucocorticoid receptor localization in human epidermal cells. Arch Dermatol Res. 1996;288:140–6.

30. Meisler N, Shull S, Xie R, Long GL, Absher M, Connolly JP, Cutroneo KR. Glucocorticoids coordinately regulate type I collagen pro alpha 1 promoter activity through both the glu-cocorticoid and transforming growth factor beta response elements: a novel mechanism of glucocorticoid regulation of eukaryotic genes. J Cell Biochem. 1995;59:376–88.

31. Nieman LK, Biller BMK, Findling JW, Newell-Price J, Savage MO, Stewart PM, Montori VM. The diagnosis of Cushing's syndrome: an Endocrine Society clinical practice guideline. J Clin Endocrinol Metab. 2008;93:1526–40.

32. Afshari A, Ardeshirpour Y, Lodish MB, et al. Facial plethora: modern Technology for Quantifying an ancient clinical sign and its use in Cushing syndrome. J Clin Endocrinol Metab. 2015;100:3928–33.

33. D'Agata R, Malozowski S, Barkan A, Cassorla F, Loriaux D. Steroid biosynthesis in human adrenal tumors. Horm Metab Res. 1987;19:386–8.

34. Mihailidis J, Dermesropian R, Taxel P, Luthra P, Grant-Kels JM. Endocrine evaluation of hirsutism. Int J Womens Dermatol. 2017;3:S6–S10.

35. Bertagna C, Orth DN. Clinical and laboratory findings and results of therapy in 58 patients with adrenocortical tumors admitted to a single medical center (1951 to 1978). Am J Med. 1981;71:855–75.

36. Thornton MJ, Hamada K, Randall VA, Messenger AG. Androgen-dependent beard dermal papilla cells secrete autocrine growth factor(s) in response to testosterone unlike scalp cells. J Invest Dermatol. 1998;111:727–32.

37. Sacerdote A, Weiss K, Tran T, Noor BR, McFarlane SI. Hypertension in patients with cushing's disease: pathophysiology, diagnosis, and management. Curr Hypertens Rep. 2005;7:212–8.

38. Klett C, Ganten D, Hellmann W, Kaling M, Ryffel GU, Weimar-Ehl T, Hackenthal E. Regulation of hepatic angiotensinogen synthesis and secretion by steroid hormones. Endocrinology. 1992;130:3660–8.

39. Saruta T, Suzuki H, Handa M, Igarashi Y, Kondo K, Senba S. Multiple factors contrib-ute to the pathogenesis of hypertension in Cushing's syndrome. J Clin Endocrinol Metab. 1986;62:275–9.

40. Isidori AM, Graziadio C, Paragliola RM, Cozzolino A, Ambrogio AG, Colao A, Corsello SM, Pivonello R. The hypertension of Cushing's syndrome: controversies in the pathophysiology and focus on cardiovascular complications. J Hypertens. 2015;33:44–60.

41. Tóth M, Grossman A. Glucocorticoid-induced osteoporosis: lessons from Cushing's syn-drome. Clin Endocrinol. 2013;79:1–11.

42. Sathyakumar S, Paul TV, Asha HS, Gnanamuthu BR, Paul MJ, Abraham DT, Rajaratnam S, Thomas N. Ectopic Cushing syndrome: a 10-year experience from a tertiary care center in southern India. Endocr Pract. 2017;23:907–14.
43. Iglesias P, Rodríguez-Berrocal V, Pian H, Díez JJ. Nelson's syndrome post-bilateral adrenalectomy. QJM Int J Med. 2016;109:561–2.
44. Gil-Cárdenas A, Herrera MF, Díaz-Polanco A, Rios JM, Pantoja JP. Nelson's syndrome after bilateral adrenalectomy for Cushing's disease. Surgery. 2007;141:147–51; discussion 151-152.
45. Klose M, Lange M, Kosteljanetz M, Poulsgaard L, Feldt-Rasmussen U. Adrenocortical insufficiency after pituitary surgery: an audit of the reliability of the conventional short synacthen test. Clin Endocrinol. 2005;63:499–505.
46. Barber TM, Adams E, Ansorge O, Byrne JV, Karavitaki N, Wass JAH. Nelson's syndrome. Eur J Endocrinol. 2010;163:495–507.
47. Barber TM, Adams E, Wass JAH. Nelson syndrome: definition and management. Handb Clin Neurol. 2014;124:327–37.
48. Patel J, Eloy JA, Liu JK. Nelson's syndrome: a review of the clinical manifestations, pathophysiology, and treatment strategies. Neurosurg Focus. 2015;38:E14.
49. Clemmons DR. Roles of insulin-like growth factor-I and growth hormone in mediating insulin resistance in acromegaly. Pituitary. 2002;5:181–3.
50. Schwartz RA. Acanthosis nigricans. J Am Acad Dermatol. 1994;31:1–19.
51. Karadağ AS, You Y, Danarti R, Al-Khuzaei S, Chen W. Acanthosis nigricans and the metabolic syndrome. Clin Dermatol. 2018;36:48–53.
52. Rudman SM, Philpott MP, Thomas GA, Kealey T. The role of IGF-I in human skin and its appendages: morphogen as well as mitogen? J Invest Dermatol. 1997;109:770–7.
53. Ben-Shlomo A, Melmed S. Skin manifestations in acromegaly. Clin Dermatol. 2006;24:256–9.
54. Chanson P, Salenave S. Acromegaly. Orphanet J Rare Dis. 2008;3:17.
55. Rick JW, Jahangiri A, Flanigan PM, Aghi MK. Patients cured of acromegaly do not experience improvement of their skull deformities. Pituitary. 2017;20:292–4.
56. Kong X, Gong S, Su L, Howard N, Kong Y. Automatic detection of acromegaly from facial photographs using machine learning methods. EBioMedicine. 2017;27:94–102.
57. Renehan AG, Shalet SM. Acromegaly and colorectal Cancer: risk assessment should be based on population-based Studiesc. J Clin Endocrinol Metab. 2002;87:1909.
58. Ben-Shlomo A, Melmed S. Acromegaly. Endocrinol Metab Clin North Am. 2008;37:101–viii.
59. Lugo G, Pena L, Cordido F. Clinical manifestations and diagnosis of acromegaly. Int J Endocrinol. 2012; https://doi.org/10.1155/2012/540398.
60. Friedrich N, Thuesen B, Jørgensen T, Juul A, Spielhagen C, Wallaschofksi H, Linneberg A. The association between IGF-I and insulin resistance: a general population study in Danish adults. Diabetes Care. 2012;35:768–73.
61. Dutta P, Bhansali A, Vaiphei K, Dutta U, Ravi Kumar P, Masoodi S, Mukherjee KK, Varma A, Kochhar R. Colonic neoplasia in acromegaly: increased proliferation or deceased apoptosis? Pituitary. 2012;15:166–73.
62. Katznelson L, Laws ER, Melmed S, Molitch ME, Murad MH, Utz A, Wass JAH. Acromegaly: an Endocrine Society clinical practice guideline. J Clin Endocrinol Metab. 2014;99:3933–51.
63. Tagliafico A, Resmini E, Nizzo R, Derchi LE, Minuto F, Giusti M, Martinoli C, Ferone D. The pathology of the ulnar nerve in acromegaly. Eur J Endocrinol. 2008;159:369–73.
64. Wiesman IM, Novak CB, Mackinnon SE, Winograd JM. Sensitivity and specificity of clinical testing for carpal tunnel syndrome. Can J Plast Surg. 2003;11:70–2.
65. Jenkins PJ, Sohaib SA, Akker S, Phillips RR, Spillane K, Wass JA, Monson JP, Grossman AB, Besser GM, Reznek RH. The pathology of median neuropathy in acromegaly. Ann Intern Med. 2000;133:197–201.
66. Sharma MD, Nguyen AV, Brown S, Robbins RJ. Cardiovascular disease in acromegaly. Methodist Debakey Cardiovasc J. 2017;13:64–7.
67. Bondanelli M, Ambrosio MR, Degli Uberti EC. Pathogenesis and prevalence of hypertension in acromegaly. Pituitary. 2001;4:239–49.

68. Kaltsas GA, Mukherjee JJ, Jenkins PJ, Satta MA, Islam N, Monson JP, Besser GM, Grossman AB. Menstrual irregularity in women with acromegaly. J Clin Endocrinol Metab. 1999;84:2731–5.
69. Dąbrowska AM, Tarach JS, Kurowska M, Nowakowski A. Thyroid diseases in patients with acromegaly. Arch Med Sci AMS. 2014;10:837–45.
70. Abreu A, Tovar AP, Castellanos R, et al. Challenges in the diagnosis and management of acromegaly: a focus on comorbidities. Pituitary. 2016;19:448–57.
71. Tahi S, Meskine D. Prolactinomas and hypogonadism in men. Clinical and developmental aspects after treatment: 21 cases. Ann Endocrinol. 2016;77:365–6.
72. Schlechte J, Sherman B, Halmi N, vanGilder J, Chapler F, Dolan K, Granner D, Duello T, Harris C. Prolactin-secreting pituitary tumors in Amenorrheic women: a comprehensive study. Endocr Rev. 1980;1:295–308.
73. Grattan DR, Jasoni CL, Liu X, Anderson GM, Herbison AE. Prolactin regulation of gonadotropin-releasing hormone neurons to suppress luteinizing hormone secretion in mice. Endocrinology. 2007;148:4344–51.
74. Glezer A, Bronstein MD. Prolactinomas. Endocrinol Metab Clin N Am. 2015;44:71–8.
75. Higuchi K, Nawata H, Maki T, Higashizima M, Kato K, Ibayashi H. Prolactin has a direct effect on adrenal androgen secretion. J Clin Endocrinol Metab. 1984;59:714–8.
76. Sakiyama R, Quan M. Galactorrhea and hyperprolactinemia. Obstet Gynecol Surv. 1983;38:689–700.
77. Chen AX, Burt MG. Hyperprolactinaemia. Aust Prescr. 2017;40:220–4.
78. Foitzik K, Langan EA, Paus R. Prolactin and the skin: a dermatological perspective on an ancient pleiotropic peptide hormone. J Invest Dermatol. 2009;129:1071–87.
79. Peli E, Satgunam P. Bitemporal hemianopia; its unique binocular complexities and a novel remedy. Ophthalmic Physiol Opt J Br Coll Ophthalmic Opt Optom. 2014;34:233–42.
80. Kedar S, Ghate D, Corbett JJ. Visual fields in neuro-ophthalmology. Indian J Ophthalmol. 2011;59:103–9.
81. Ogra S, Nichols AD, Stylli S, Kaye AH, Savino PJ, Danesh-Meyer HV. Visual acuity and pattern of visual field loss at presentation in pituitary adenoma. J Clin Neurosci Off J Neurosurg Soc Australas. 2014;21:735–40.
82. Schmalisch K, Milian M, Schimitzek T, Lagrèze WA, Honegger J. Predictors for visual dysfunction in nonfunctioning pituitary adenomas - implications for neurosurgical management. Clin Endocrinol. 2012;77:728–34.
83. Gan L, Ma J, Feng F, et al. The predictive value of Suprasellar extension for visual function evaluation in Chinese patients with nonfunctioning pituitary adenoma with optic chiasm compression. World Neurosurg. 2018;116:e960–7.
84. Lee IH, Miller NR, Zan E, Tavares F, Blitz AM, Sung H, Yousem DM, Boland MV. Visual defects in patients with pituitary adenomas: the myth of Bitemporal Hemianopsia. Am J Roentgenol. 2015;205:W512–8.
85. Sperling S, Bhatt H. Prolactinoma: a massive effect on bone mineral density in a young patient. Case Rep Endocrinol. 2016; https://doi.org/10.1155/2016/6312621.
86. Beshyah SA, Freemantle C, Thomas E, Rutherford O, Page B, Murphy M, Johnston DG. Abnormal body composition and reduced bone mass in growth hormone deficient hypopituitary adults. Clin Endocrinol. 1995;42:179–89.
87. Binnerts A, Deurenberg P, Swart GR, Wilson JH, Lamberts SW. Body composition in growth hormone-deficient adults. Am J Clin Nutr. 1992;55:918–23.
88. Johansen T, Richelsen B, Hansen HS, Din N, Malmlöf K. Growth hormone-mediated breakdown of body fat: effects of GH on lipases in adipose tissue and skeletal muscle of old rats fed different diets. Horm Metab Res Horm Stoffwechselforschung Horm Metab. 2003;35:243–50.
89. Frayn KN, Coppack SW, Fielding BA, Humphreys SM. Coordinated regulation of hormone-sensitive lipase and lipoprotein lipase in human adipose tissue in vivo: implications for the control of fat storage and fat mobilization. Adv Enzym Regul. 1995;35:163–78.

90. Chaves VE, Júnior FM, Bertolini GL. The metabolic effects of growth hormone in adipose tissue. Endocrine. 2013;44:293–302.
91. Møller N, Copeland KC, Nair KS. Growth hormone effects on protein metabolism. Endocrinol Metab Clin N Am. 2007;36:89–100.
92. Khan R, Jehangir W, Regeti K, Yousif A. Hypertriglyceridemia-induced pancreatitis: choice of treatment. Gastroenterol Res. 2015;8:234–6.
93. Díez JJ, Sangiao-Alvarellos S, Cordido F. Treatment with growth hormone for adults with growth hormone deficiency syndrome: benefits and risks. Int J Mol Sci. 2018; https://doi.org/10.3390/ijms19030893.
94. Kurtoğlu S, Hatipoglu N. Growth hormone insensitivity: diagnostic and therapeutic approaches. J Endocrinol Investig. 2016;39:19–28.
95. Castilla-Cortazar I, Ita JRD, Aguirre GA, Rodríguez-Rivera J, García-Magariño M, Martín-Estal I, Flores-Caloca Ó, Diaz-Olachea C. Primary growth hormone insensitivity and psychomotor delay. Clin Case Rep. 2018;6:426–31.
96. Janecka A, Kołodziej-Rzepa M, Biesaga B. Clinical and molecular features of Laron syndrome, a genetic disorder protecting from Cancer. Vivo Athens Greece. 2016;30:375–81.
97. Ohlsson C, Bengtsson B-Å, Isaksson OGP, Andreassen TT, Slootweg MC. Growth hormone and bone. Endocr Rev. 1998;19:55–79.
98. Laron Z. Insulin-like growth factor 1 (IGF-1): a growth hormone. Mol Pathol. 2001;54:311–6.
99. Lindsey RC, Mohan S. Skeletal effects of growth hormone and insulin-like growth factor-I therapy. Mol Cell Endocrinol. 2016;432:44–55.
100. Long F, Ornitz DM. Development of the endochondral skeleton. Cold Spring Harb Perspect Biol. 2013;5:a008334.
101. Nilsson O, Marino R, De Luca F, Phillip M, Baron J. Endocrine regulation of the growth plate. Horm Res. 2005;64:157–65.
102. Lui JC, Nilsson O, Baron J. Recent research on the growth plate: recent insights into the regulation of the growth plate. J Mol Endocrinol. 2014;53:T1–9.
103. Ginsberg S, Laron Z, Bed MA, Vaisman N. The obesity of patients with Laron syndrome is not associated with excessive nutritional intake. Obes Res Clin Pract. 2009;3:1–52.
104. Laron Z. Laron syndrome (primary growth hormone resistance or insensitivity): the personal experience 1958–2003. J Clin Endocrinol Metab. 2004;89:1031–44.
105. Velloso CP. Regulation of muscle mass by growth hormone and IGF-I. Br J Pharmacol. 2008;154:557–68.
106. Cotta OR, Santarpia L, Curtò L, Aimaretti G, Corneli G, Trimarchi F, Cannavò S. Primary growth hormone insensitivity (Laron syndrome) and acquired hypothyroidism: a case report. J Med Case Rep. 2011;5:301.
107. Griffeth RJ, Bianda V, Nef S. The emerging role of insulin-like growth factors in testis development and function. Basic Clin Androl. 2014;24:12.
108. Guevara-Aguirre J, Balasubramanian P, Guevara-Aguirre M, et al. Growth hormone receptor deficiency is associated with a major reduction in pro-aging signaling, Cancer and diabetes in humans. Sci Transl Med. 2011;3:70ra13.
109. Denduluri SK, Idowu O, Wang Z, et al. Insulin-like growth factor (IGF) signaling in tumorigenesis and the development of cancer drug resistance. Genes Dis. 2015;2:13–25.
110. Guevara-Aguirre J, Rosenbloom AL. Obesity, diabetes and cancer: insight into the relationship from a cohort with growth hormone receptor deficiency. Diabetologia. 2015;58:37–42.
111. Nakamichi A, Ocho K, Oka K, Yasuda M, Hasegawa K, Iwamuro M, Obika M, Rai K, Otsuka F. Manifestation of central diabetes insipidus in a patient with thyroid storm. Intern Med Tokyo Jpn. 2018;57:1939–42.
112. Boone M, Deen PMT. Physiology and pathophysiology of the vasopressin-regulated renal water reabsorption. Pflugers Arch. 2008;456:1005–24.
113. Oksche A, Rosenthal W. The molecular basis of nephrogenic diabetes insipidus. J Mol Med Berl Ger. 1998;76:326–37.

114. Moritz ML, Ayus JC. Chapter 8 - diabetes insipidus and syndrome of inappropriate antidiuretic hormone. In: Singh AK, Williams GH, editors. Textb. Nephro-Endocrinol. 2nd ed: Academic Press; 2018. p. 133–61.
115. Park KS, Yoo KY. Role of vasopressin in current anesthetic practice. Korean J Anesthesiol. 2017;70:245–57.
116. Loh JA, Verbalis JG. Disorders of water and salt metabolism associated with pituitary disease. Endocrinol Metab Clin N Am. 2008;37:213–34.
117. Verrua E, Mantovani G, Ferrante E, Noto A, Sala E, Malchiodi E, Iapichino G, Peccoz PB, Spada A. Severe water intoxication secondary to the concomitant intake of non-steroidal anti-inflammatory drugs and desmopressin: a case report and review of the literature. Horm Athens Greece. 2013;12:135–41.
118. Li Y, Wei Y, Zheng F, Guan Y, Zhang X. Prostaglandin E2 in the regulation of water transport in renal collecting ducts. Int J Mol Sci. 2017; https://doi.org/10.3390/ijms18122539.
119. Gao M, Cao R, Du S, et al. Disruption of prostaglandin E2 receptor EP4 impairs urinary concentration via decreasing aquaporin 2 in renal collecting ducts. Proc Natl Acad Sci. 2015;112:8397–402.

Thyroid Gland Signs

2

Learning Objectives
At the end of this chapter, you will be able to:

1. Understand the metabolic effects of active thyroid hormone in various tissues in the human body
2. Understand the pathophysiologic basis for the classic clinical signs of Graves' disease
3. Recognize how the anatomical relations of the thyroid gland explains compressive clinical signs in the setting of goiters
4. Understand the pathophysiologic basis of thyroid hormone resistance.

2.1 Hashimoto's Thyroiditis

2.1.1 Queen Anne's Sign

Clinical Features

This eponymous medical sign is named after Anne of Denmark, due to her truncated lateral eyebrows, which was depicted in a portrait by Paul Van Somer [1]. Facial and body hair tends to be dry, thin, and brittle in hypothyroidism. Loss of hair over the lateral third of the eyebrow is a recognized sign of hypothyroidism [2].

Pathophysiology

1. Triiodothyronine (T3) and tetraiodothyronine (T4) have direct effects on the human scalp. T3 and T4 both play essential roles in hair follicle growth, apoptosis, and keratin expression. T4 prolongs the growth phase of the hair follicle (anagen). This, in part, explains the reason for telogen effluvium in hypothyroid patients [3].

© Springer Nature Switzerland AG 2020
A. Manni, A. Quarde, *Endocrine Pathophysiology*,
https://doi.org/10.1007/978-3-030-49872-6_2

2. Lack of expression of keratin due to low T4 levels accounts for the thin and brittle hair follicles in hypothyroid patients [3].

Conditions which May Present with Queen Anne's Sign
Queen Anne's sign is also known as Hertoghe's sign. It may be seen in a myriad of other medical conditions, including syphilis [4], leprosy, atopic dermatitis, seborrheic dermatitis, psoriasis, and biotin deficiency, to name a few [5].

2.1.2   Bradycardia

Clinical Features
Hypothyroidism is a known cause of bradycardia and significant bradyarrhythmias such as high-grade atrioventricular (AV) block. A recent retrospective study involving 668 subjects reported the need for permanent pacemaker insertions in some patients who presented with high-grade AV block, even after resolution of hypothyroidism [6].

Pathophysiology
T3 increases atrial myocyte pacemaker current frequency by improving the function of the sodium-calcium exchanger. This has been demonstrated in animal models. The mechanism underlying the cause of bradycardia has, however, not been elucidated in humans [7, 8].

2.1.3   Pericardial and Pleural Effusions

Clinical Features
The incidence of pericardial effusions ranges between 3 and 6%, in mainly advanced stages of hypothyroidism. Pericardial effusions in mild hypothyroidism are, however, rare [9, 10]. Pleural effusion can be diagnosed by eliciting a "stony dull" percussion note and reduced tactile vocal fremitus over the lung zones [11]. Distant heart sounds, hypotension [12], pulsus paradoxus, and jugular venous distension may be observed in significant pericardial effusions [13].

Pathophysiology
There is a substantial increase in the extravascular content of albumin due to the transcapillary escape of albumin [14, 15]. Compensatory fractional return of extravasated fluid via the lymphatic system, in response to "albumin leak," is impaired in hypothyroidism due to the accumulation of mucopolysaccharide protein complexes in the interstitial space. The response to this based on Starling's forces is the retention of extravascular fluid, which can manifest as pleural and pericardial effusions [14].

2.1.4 Dry Skin

Clinical Features
Dry skin (xerosis) is a cardinal skin manifestation of hypothyroidism [16]. Xerosis is the most frequent cutaneous manifestation of hypothyroidism, with a prevalence greater than 65% [17]. In a small study designed to assess the predictive value of the physical examination in suggesting a diagnosis of hypothyroidism, rough, dry skin had a reported positive likelihood ratio (+LR) of +2.3 in diagnosing hypothyroidism [18].

Pathophysiology
There are thyroid hormone receptors present in the skin and its appendages; as such, perturbations in thyroid hormone levels result in various skin manifestations [16, 19].

1. Diminished sebaceous gland units reduce the extent of dermal secretions [19]. Sweat glands in significant hypothyroidism are atrophic due to a yet to be elucidated mechanism [16].
2. Reduced epidermal sterol synthesis produces dryness of the hypothyroid skin [19].

Other cutaneous changes seen in clinically significant hypothyroidism include lymphedema and myxedema (Table 2.1).

2.1.5 Macroglossia

Clinical Features
Macroglossia is a rare sign of hypothyroidism [21] and is described as protrusion of the tongue beyond the teeth during a state of normal relaxation of the tongue musculature [22].

Pathophysiology
Dysregulation in the formation of hydrophilic glycosaminoglycans leads to their accumulation in the interstitium [23]. As was previously described for hypothyroidism induced-pericardial effusions, there is an accumulation of extravascular fluid in various tissues, including those of the tongue [14, 23] (see Sect. 2.1.3).

Table 2.1 Other skin manifestations of hypothyroidism

Lesion	Pathophysiology
Lymphedema (hands, face, and eyelids)	Accumulation of hydrophilic mucopolysaccharides in the interstitial space impairs lymphatic drainage [20]
Myxedema	Deposition of mucopolysaccharides in the skin [20]

Adapted from Ai et al. [20]

2.1.6 Hyporeflexia

Clinical Features

Hyporeflexia in hypothyroidism classically presents as a delayed relaxation phase of deep tendon reflexes (DTRs) [24]. This has been eponymously labeled as the "Woltman's sign of myxedema" [25]. It is best elicited at the ankle joint with the patient in a seated position and the lower extremities in a dependent position. This allows an accurate assessment of the relaxation phase of the reflex since relaxation will be occurring against gravity [26].

Pathophysiology

Decreased myosin calcium-ATPase activity, with a concomitantly reduced rate of sequestration of calcium in the sarcoplasmic reticulum of the skeletal muscle, accounts for Woltman's sign [27]. T3 plays a critical role in muscle metabolism through its effects on the sarcoplasmic reticulum Calcium-ATPase function. Prolonged skeletal muscle contraction occurs due to impaired sequestration of calcium by the sarcoplasmic reticulum in the setting of low T3. This increases the duration of the relaxation phase of DTRs [28].

2.1.7 Proximal Myopathy

Clinical Features

Myopathy presents with proximal muscle weakness involving the pelvic or shoulder girdle musculature [29]. Clinically identifiable neuromuscular dysfunction had a prevalence of approximately 40% in a prospective cohort study assessing neuromuscular dysfunction in patients with hypothyroidism [30].

Hoffman syndrome, a form of hypothyroid-related muscular dysfunction, is described as a triad of *muscle weakness*, *hyporeflexia*, and *muscular hypertrophy* [31].

Pathophysiology

Low levels of T4 impair glycogen breakdown in skeletal muscle and contributes to selective atrophy of fast-twitch type 2 skeletal muscle fibers [29]. This leads to a state of a predominance of slow-twitch type 1 skeletal muscle fibers, which results in the weakness observed in subjects with hypothyroidism [32, 33].

2.1.8 Galactorrhea

Clinical Features

Patients may present with galactorrhea, although spontaneous or expressible galactorrhea is a rare finding in primary hypothyroidism [34].

Pathophysiology

- Low circulating levels of free T3, as occurs in primary hypothyroidism, results in a loss of feedback inhibition of T3 on TRH producing cells of the hypothalamus. This is followed by the release of TRH, which has a stimulatory effect on pituitary lactotrophs, resulting in increased production of prolactin from the anterior pituitary. Prolactin stimulates glandular breast tissue proliferation, leading to galactorrhea.
- Additionally, there is also a loss of negative feedback inhibition of lactotrophs by T3. This compounds the state of excess prolactin secretion.
- Reduced metabolic clearance of prolactin (PRL) due to hypothyroidism contributes to high circulating levels of prolactin.
- Finally, TRH stimulation of both thyrotropes and lactotrophs promotes pituitary hyperplasia. Enlargement of the pituitary gland causes a "stalk effect," which blocks the dopaminergic tracts involved in reducing lactotroph production of PRL [35] (see Fig. 2.1).

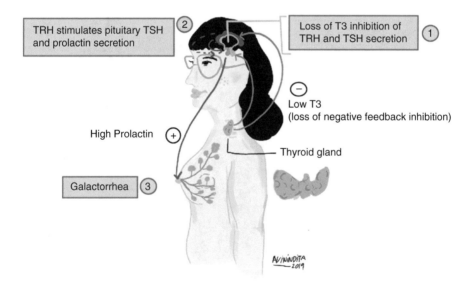

Fig. 2.1   Schematic diagram depicting the pathophysiologic basis of hyperprolactinemia in primary hypothyroidism. Low circulating levels of active thyroid hormone (T3) results in a loss of negative feedback inhibition of both hypothalamic and pituitary thyrotropin-releasing hormone (TRH) and thyroid-stimulating hormone (TSH) release, respectively (step 1). Increased TRH secretion, in turn, stimulates both pituitary lactotrophs and thyrotrophs (step 2). Also, inadequate clearance of prolactin due to hypothyroidism-induced hypometabolism contributes to hyperprolactinemia and galactorrhea (step 3) [35]. (Based on Ansari et al. [35])

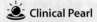 **Clinical Pearl**

Pituitary Pseudotumor

Thyrotrope hyperplasia (pituitary pseudotumor) can occur in patients with a long-standing history of primary hypothyroidism. It is a condition that is entirely reversible with timely initiation of thyroid hormone replacement [36]. The diagnosis of primary hypothyroidism should be considered in patients with diffuse enlargement of the pituitary gland, without an obvious adenoma, in the setting of hyperprolactinemia [37].

 Questions You Might Be Asked on Rounds

What is the reason for yellowing of the skin in some hypothyroid patients?

Yellowing of the skin is due to hypercarotenemia, and it tends to involve the palms, soles of the feet, and nasolabial folds. A reduction in hepatic metabolism of β-carotene accounts for its excess circulating levels. β-Carotene is subsequently deposited in the skin, and this results in the characteristic yellowish hue of the skin [20].

Why would a patient with Hashimoto's thyroiditis develop eye and skin changes somewhat like Graves' disease?

Cross-reactivity between circulating anti-thyroid peroxidase antibodies and fibroblasts present in the orbit and skin [20].

Besides, some patients with Hashimoto's thyroiditis have increased thyroid-stimulating immunoglobulins (TSI) as well, which may contribute to eye and dermal manifestations similar to Graves' disease. Autoimmune thyroid disease is a balance between thyroid hormone-blocking and stimulating antibodies. The antibody which predominates determines the disorder, i.e., Hashimoto's thyroiditis or Graves' disease. At any point in the disorder, the balance may change [38].

2.2   Graves' Disease

2.2.1   Thyroid Eye Disease

Clinical Features

Thyroid eye disease (TED) is the most common extra-thyroidal manifestation of Graves' disease [39]. TED can present with a myriad of ocular signs, including photophobia, proptosis, or conjunctival injection [40]. Other signs suggestive of TED include lid lag, globe lag, lid retraction, and even, in some severe cases, evidence of optic neuropathy [41].

Table 2.2 Selected eponymous thyroid eye signs in Graves' disease

Eye sign	Clinical findings
Dalrymple's sign	Lid retraction involving the upper eyelid [45]
Von Grafe's sign	Lagging of the upper eyelid upon downward gaze [45]
Collier's sign	Lid retraction involving the lower eyelid [45]
Stellwag's sign	Infrequent blinking of the eyelids [45, 46]
Rosenbach's sign	Tremors of the eyelids upon closure [46]
Gifford sign	A difficulty with eversion of the upper eyelids [46]
Jellinek sign	Hyperpigmentation of the upper eyelids [46]
Sainton sign	Nystagmus on the voluntary horizontal movement of the eyes [46]
Ballet sign	Paresis of extraocular muscles [46]
Enroth sign	Periorbital edema [46]
Griffith's sign	Lid lag involving the lower eyelid on upward gaze [46]

Adapted from references Mallika [45] and Urrets-Zavalia [46]

Pathophysiology
- Orbital fibroblasts have TSH and IGF-1 receptors, which are directly stimulated by thyroid-stimulating immunoglobulins (TSIs). There is an enhanced proliferation of orbital fibroblasts as a consequence, which eventually causes extensive fibrosis in the orbit [42]. *Teprotumumab*, a monoclonal antibody that targets the IGF-1 receptor, was recently approved for the management of TED. Teprotumumab resulted in a significant reduction in proptosis, clinical activity score, and diplopia when compared to placebo [43].
- TSI also mediates the differentiation of orbital fibroblasts into adipocytes and myofibroblasts. A state of hyperproliferation of adipocytes and myofibroblasts increases periorbital soft tissue volume [44].
- Also, orbital fibroblasts exhibit an exaggerated inflammatory response in the setting of TSI-TSH receptor interaction. There is an accumulation of extracellular matrix in the setting of this pro-inflammatory milieu, which leads to soft tissue edema and proptosis [40, 41].

There are a host of thyroid eye signs named after the clinicians who first described them. A few have been outlined in Table 2.2.

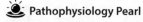 **Pathophysiology Pearl**

Why do patients with Graves' disease have upper eyelid retraction?

- Muller's muscle (superior tarsal muscle) under the sympathetic stimulation of excess circulating thyroid hormones contracts and contributes to lid retraction [47].
- Due to extensive orbital inflammation, the levator palpebrae superioris is infiltrated by inflammatory cells, which leads to fibrosis and contraction of the muscle [47].
- Although lid retraction occurs in Graves' disease, it is not pathognomonic for this condition and can occur in other forms of hyperthyroidism [48].

2.2.2   Pretibial Myxedema

Clinical Features

Pretibial myxedema (PM) is a cutaneous manifestation of Graves' disease and can appear as non-pitting edema, plaque-like, or nodular lesions. In severe cases, it may appear like the lymphedema associated with elephantiasis. The nodular variant occurs in fewer than 10% of subjects and has been reported to mimic the characteristic lesions of erythema nodosum [49]. PM can recur several years after definitive treatment of Graves' disease, i.e., surgery or radioactive iodine ablation [50].

Pathophysiology

The exact mechanism has not been elucidated at this time, although the lesions are noted to be present at sites of repetitive trauma. The influx of inflammatory cells and fibroblast proliferation have been proposed as possible reasons for pretibial myxedema. Histologically, there is an accumulation of mucopolysaccharides in the dermis of the skin [49], and the process is believed to be mediated by circulating TSI acting on TSH receptors present on fibroblasts in the skin [51, 52].

Other cutaneous manifestations of hyperthyroidism include urticaria, telangiectasia, erythema, and warm skin (Table 2.3).

2.2.3   Thyroid Acropachy

Clinical Features

Thyroid acropachy (TA) is characterized by digital clubbing involving the upper and lower extremity digits. It has a strong association with thyroid eye disease [58, 59] and may, in some instances, herald a diagnosis of Graves' disease [60].

Pathophysiology

Accumulation of glycosaminoglycans and concomitant fibroblast proliferation have also been proposed as the underlying mechanisms of thyroid acropachy [59].

Table 2.3   Other skin manifestations of hyperthyroidism

Lesion	Pathophysiology
Warm and moist skin	Vasodilation of cutaneous vessels [53]
Palmar erythema	Vasodilation of cutaneous vessels [54, 55]
Urticaria	Binding of anti-TPO immunoglobulin E antibodies to receptors on the surface of mast cells leads to their activation and degranulation [56]
Telangiectasia	Increased dermal blood flow and a possible immune-mediated process have been proposed [57]

TPO thyroid peroxidase
Adapted from references [53–57]

Clinical Pearl

What might be seen on a plain radiograph of an involved extremity, for patients with TA?

A periosteal reaction involving bones of the hand or feet might be seen on a plain radiograph. TA presents with a clinical triad of periosteal reaction, swelling of the hands or feet, and clubbing of the digits [60].

2.2.4 Onycholysis

Clinical Features
Onycholysis has eponymously been referred to as "Plummer's nails." Dr. Henry Plummer of Mayo Clinic described various characteristic features of dystrophic nails in hyperthyroidism, including the unique "scoop shovel" appearance and flattening of the fingernails [61]. Plummer's nails present as a separation of the distal aspect of the nail from its underlying nail bed. It is an inconsistent physical finding and occurs in approximately 5% of patients with hyperthyroidism [62].

Pathophysiology
The cause of onycholysis remains unclear, although hyperthyroidism-induced catabolism and rapid growth of the underlying nail bed are possible reasons for separation of the nail from the nail bed [63].

2.2.5 Periodic Paralysis

Clinical Features
A form of periodic paralysis known as thyrotoxic periodic paralysis (TPP) occurs in patients with Graves' disease and may present with either mild muscle weakness or overt flaccid paresis [64]. TPP presents most often in people of East Asian descent but has been described in other ethnicities [65].

Pathophysiology
- T3 enters the mitochondria of skeletal muscle cells and increases metabolism with subsequent generation of ATP. ATP increases the activity of sodium-potassium ATPase present in skeletal muscle [66] and promotes an increase in the transcellular shift of potassium, which results in hyperpolarization of the skeletal cell membrane. Hyperpolarized skeletal muscle tissue has reduced excitability, and this accounts for reduced muscular contraction and paralysis [67].
- T3 also increases gene expression and subsequent translation of the sodium-potassium ATPase. The increased presence and subsequent enhanced activation of the sodium-potassium ATPase in skeletal muscle contributes to TPP [67].

2.2.6   Thyroid Bruit and Thrill

Clinical Features

Bruits auscultated over the superior thyroid arteries are detectable in up to 85% of patients with symptomatic hyperthyroidism. They are continuous (throughout the cardiac cycle) and are accentuated in the systolic phase of the cardiac cycle [68]. The auscultatory findings of a thyroid bruit are different from those of carotid bruits or radiating cardiac murmurs to the neck. The bruit associated with carotid artery disease, for example, tends to occur only in the systolic phase of the cardiac cycle [69].

It is worthy to note that the presence of a thyroid bruit on the clinical exam is pathognomonic for an autonomously hyperfunctioning gland (Graves' disease). This clinical finding effectively rules out thyroiditis in patients with biochemical hyperthyroidism [70].

Pathophysiology

Hyperthyroidism-mediated accelerated blood flow accounts for the continuous bruit heard over the superior thyroid arteries [68].

2.2.7   Tachycardia

Clinical Features

Patients with hyperthyroidism classically have tachycardia, with more than 90% having a resting heart rate higher than 90 beats per minute [71]. Atrial fibrillation, a cause of tachycardia, is, however, less frequent in Graves' disease. Indeed, elderly patients with "apathetic hyperthyroidism" are more likely to have atrial fibrillation than younger patients [53]. An irregularly irregular peripheral pulse is a hallmark of atrial fibrillation on the clinical exam [72].

Pathophysiology

- Triiodothyronine (T3) increases the duration of activation of myocardial sodium channels, which leads to increased intracellular sodium. An increased intracellular sodium concentration then stimulates the *sodium-calcium antiport system*, which is critical in maintaining intramyocardial calcium concentrations. Accentuated sodium-calcium antiport activity increases intramyocardial calcium and promotes myocardial contractility [73].
- T3 upregulates the β1 adrenergic receptor expression not only in the myocardium but also in the Juxtaglomerular cells (JGCs) of the kidney. Catecholamine activation of β1 receptors of the JGCs is responsible for the release of renin and eventual activation of the renin-angiotensin-aldosterone system (RAAS)(see Fig. 3.1). Sodium and fluid retention increases cardiac preload and contractility (Frank-Starling law of the heart) [73].

- T3 binds to intracellular thyroid hormone response elements involved in the transcription and translation of *calcium adenosine triphosphatase (Ca-ATPase)* in the myocardial sarcoplasmic reticulum. Ca-ATPase is essential in regulating intramuscular calcium concentration. An increase in myocardial calcium concentration accounts for the exaggerated inotropic effects of excess T3 [7].
- T3 increases myocardial calcium uptake through direct activation of the myocardial L-type calcium channels. This contributes to the inotropic effect of thyroid hormone excess [71].
- The upregulation of a myocardial gap junction protein critical in the transmission of electrical impulses has been proposed as a mechanism of hyperthyroidism-induced atrial fibrillation [74].
- The effects of T3 include a blunting of cardiac parasympathetic tone and an increase in tissue sensitivity to the effects of normal circulating catecholamines [75].

2.2.8 Gynecomastia

Clinical Features
Gynecomastia is a known clinical manifestation of thyrotoxicosis but is seldom a presenting feature of the disease. Gynecomastia is usually reversible after the control of hyperthyroidism [76]. It presents as palpable subareolar tissue and should be differentiated from pseudogynecomastia (lipomastia), which is a generalized accumulation of fat in male breasts [77, 78].

Pathophysiology
- Thyroid hormone increases the synthesis of sex hormone-binding globulin (SHBG) by the liver. SHBG binds to testosterone and reduces the circulating level of free testosterone (active or unbound testosterone). A significant lowering of the *androgen/estrogen ratio* promotes mammary gland proliferation due to the effects of estrogen [78].
- Increased peripheral aromatization of androgens into estrogens [78].

2.2.9 Lymphadenopathy

Clinical Features
Perithyroidal lymphadenopathy is a reported finding in benign thyroid disease. Up to a third of patients with Graves' disease in a recent cross-sectional study were noted to have clinically discernible perithyroidal lymph node enlargement [79].

Pathophysiology
Reactive lymphocyte proliferation (lymphoid hyperplasia) in the setting of autoimmune thyroiditis [80]

2.2.10 Change in Body Composition (Weight Loss)

Clinical Features

Patients with uncontrolled thyrotoxicosis present with unintentional weight loss in the setting of hyperphagia. Loss of body fat and muscle bulk may be discernible on the routine clinical examination [81].

Pathophysiology
- Resting energy expenditure (REE) is a critical determinant of weight and is dependent on brown adipose tissue (BAT) mitochondrial activity. In stark contrast to the role of mitochondria in other tissues, BAT mitochondria are not primarily involved in ATP generation. They possess an uncoupling protein that interrupts the electron transport chain and allows the transduction of mitochondrial membrane potential energy directly into heat energy [82]. T3 increases thermogenesis in brown adipose tissue by potentiating the effects of the uncoupling protein involved in the BAT mitochondrial electron transport chain [81].
- Type 2 deiodinase enzyme activity (involved in the peripheral conversion of free T4 into free T3) is also upregulated in BAT. This increases the local concentration of T3, further compounding the effects of T3 on the mitochondrial uncoupling protein [81].

 Pathophysiology Pearl

Thyroid hormone synthesis (Fig. 2.2)

 Questions You Might Be Asked on Rounds

What is the mechanism underlying cutaneous hyperpigmentation seen in Graves' disease?

Hyperthyroxinemia leads to accelerated metabolism of cortisol. Low serum cortisol causes a compensatory increase in adrenocorticotrophic hormone (ACTH) due to the loss of negative feedback inhibition of cortisol on ACTH production. ACTH mediates hyperpigmentation of the skin (see Sect. 3.1.2) [20]. This proposed mechanism of increased cortisol metabolism may explain a rare report of adrenal crisis in a hyperthyroid patient with cryptic, non-classic 21-hydroxylase deficiency [84].

Why may pretibial myxedema not improve after treatment of Graves' disease?

Treatment of Graves' disease with thyroidectomy or radioactive iodine ablation does not prevent the production of thyroid-stimulating immunoglobulins (TSIs). Circulating TSIs can still stimulate TSH receptors present on dermal fibroblasts long after the cure of hyperthyroidism [85].

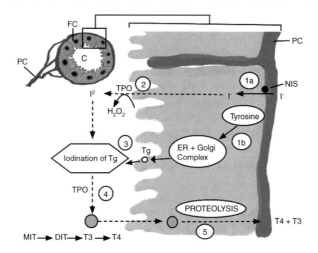

Fig. 2.2 Synthesis of T3 and T4 by the thyroid follicular unit. Iodide(I⁻) is transported from the perifollicular capillary (PC) into the thyroid follicular cell (FC) by the basal sodium-iodide symporter (NIS), under a sodium electrochemical gradient facilitated by the sodium-potassium pump (step 1a). Thyroglobulin (Tg) is synthesized from tyrosine residues, a process that occurs in the rough endoplasmic reticulum (step 1b). Tg undergoes further posttranslational modification in the Golgi apparatus of the follicular cell. It is then secreted into the follicular lumen (site of colloid storage) through a process of exocytosis. Iodide is transported to the apical membrane of the thyroid follicular cell, where thyroid peroxidase (TPO) enzyme catalyzes the oxidation of iodide to iodine. This oxidation step requires hydrogen peroxide(H_2O_2)(step 2). Tyrosyl residues on the thyroglobulin molecule undergo iodination by the previously oxidized iodine molecule. This process of "organification" is facilitated by TPO and results in the formation of monoiodothyronine (MIT) and diiodiothyronine (DIT) residues (step 3). Triiodothyronine (T3) and tetraiodothyronine (T4) are then formed in a final coupling reaction which involves the formation of ester linkages between "donor" and "acceptor" iodothyronine (MIT or DIT) residues (step 4). The thyroid follicular cell ingests colloid (C) by pinocytosis through the apical membrane. Proteolysis of the colloidal substrate in the thyroid follicular cell yields thyroglobulin, MIT, DIT, T3, and T4 (step 5). Deiodinases present in the follicular cell convert some T4 into active thyroid hormone (T3). Thyroid hormones (T3 and T4) are then actively transported across the basolateral plasma membrane of the thyroid epithelial cell into capillary [83]. (Based on Carvalho et al. [83])

2.3   Euthyroid Goiter with Thoracic Outlet Syndrome

2.3.1   Pemberton's Sign

Clinical Features
This sign is eponymously named after Dr. Hugh Pemberton, who described this classic physical finding in a letter published in Lancet in 1946 titled "sign of a submerged goitre." He explained the method of eliciting the sign, expected clinical findings, and also proposed a mechanism for the physical finding [86].

The sign is elicited by instructing the patient to lift their arms such that the arms touch both sides of the head. The patient is then instructed to hold their arms in that position until facial congestion or erythema is noticed [86].

Pathophysiology
In a recent case report, magnetic resonance imaging (MRI) of the neck was used to elucidate the mechanism underlying Pemberton's sign. In this report of a patient with a retrosternal goiter, there was no demonstrable craniocaudal change in the position of the thyroid gland during the maneuver to elicit the sign. The widely accepted "cork effect" initially proposed by Pemberton was not consistent with the MRI findings noted in the study. The authors objectively confirmed compression of the external jugular and subclavian veins by the clavicles during the clinical maneuver. The thoracic inlet, however, remained relatively fixed in size, thus discounting the "cork effect" as a plausible explanation of Pemberton's sign [87].

2.3.2   Other Compressive Signs (Superior Vena Cava Syndrome, Phrenic Nerve Paralysis)

Clinical Features
Superior vena cava (SVC) syndrome can occur in patients with large goiters. There are multiple case reports of mediastinal goiters leading to SVC syndrome. A goiter may sometimes not be palpable on the physical exam due to its ectopic position in the mediastinum [88–90].

Clinically significant dyspnea due to either unilateral or bilateral phrenic nerve compression by large retrosternal goiters has been reported [91, 92]. In a recent large series of 50 retrosternal goiters, nerve compression syndromes were second only to tracheal compression in terms of clinically significant complications [93].

Pathophysiology
The compression of the brachiocephalic vessels by an extrinsic retrosternal thyroidal mass causes SVC syndrome. Ipsilateral distension of the subclavian, axillary, and jugular veins occurs as a consequence of impaired drainage of the brachiocephalic veins [90].

The phrenic nerve supplies motor innervation to the diaphragm and is derived from the 3rd, 4th, and 5th cervical nerves and passes in front of the anterior scalene muscle on its descent from the neck into the thoracic cavity [94, 95]. Extrinsic compression of the phrenic nerve during either its intrathoracic or cervical course results in dyspnea [92] (Table 2.4).

Table 2.4   Modified World Health Organization (WHO) classification for the clinical evaluation of a goiter

Grade	Examination findings
Grade 0	Goiter not visible or palpable [96, 97]
Grade 1	Goiter not visible in the normal position of the neck but is palpable. The thyroidal mass should be palpable on deglutition [96, 97]
Grade 2	Visible and palpable goiter [96, 97]

Adapted from references Lewinski [96] and Abuye [97]

Pathophysiology Pearl

Pathogenesis of nodular goiter formation [98]

- There is an initial insult to the thyroid in the form of nutritional iodine deficiency, goitrogens, or even autoimmune thyroid disease, which results in reduced thyroid hormone synthesis.
- As an adaptation to decreased active thyroid hormone, there is a reduction in negative feedback inhibition of the central thyrotropes, causing an increase in TSH stimulation of thyroid follicular cells. Thyroid hyperplasia and hydrogen peroxide generated as a result of hypermetabolism increase the risk of genetic mutations. This high replication rate reduces the time for the repair of possible mutations, leading to persistent errors in transcription and translation of deoxyribonucleic acid (DNA).
- Some of the mistakes (gain-of-function mutations) involve the constitutive intrathyroidal cyclic adenosine monophosphate pathways (TSH receptor), which further promotes excessive clonal proliferation.
- Continuous clonal expansion contributes to additional mutations, which may result in the formation of "hot" or "cold" nodules [98].

 Questions You Might Be Asked on Rounds

What is Riedel's thyroiditis?

It is a rare fibrosclerosing condition of the thyroid, characterized by a "stony hard" thyroid consistency. Involvement of thyrocervical tissues leads to a change in voice (recurrent laryngeal nerve infiltration) and other compressive symptoms such as dysphagia and dyspnea [99]. *Riedel's thyroiditis* is now appreciated as a thyroidal manifestation of *IgG4-related systemic disease* (IgG4-RSD) [100]. IgG4-RSD has an unclear etiology, although a predominant lymphoplasmacytic infiltrate and elevated serum IgG4 (immunoglobulin G4) are hallmarks of this disease. Extra-thyroidal involvement of sialolacrimal glands, hepatobiliary system, and retroperitoneum have been reported [101].

How does thyromegaly result in Horner's syndrome? (Fig. 2.3).

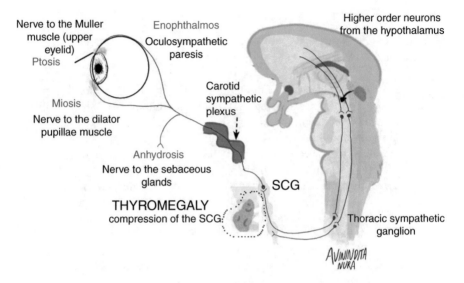

Fig. 2.3 Pathogenesis of thyromegaly induced Horner's syndrome. Horner's syndrome classically presents with ptosis, miosis, and enophthalmos. The superior cervical ganglion (SCG) serves as a relay center for higher-order neurons and has projecting from it, postganglionic neurons, which will eventually terminate in the orbit, skin of the head and neck region [102, 103]. The SCG lies near the thyroid and is subject to extrinsic compression in the setting of significant thyromegaly [104]. Distal innervation of Muller's muscle, dilator pupillae muscle, and sebaceous glands in the skin can be impaired by clinically significant thyromegaly (compression of the SCG). Motor neurons supplying Muller's muscle are involved, accounting for ptosis. The involvement of sympathetic innervation of the dilator pupillae muscle accounts for miosis. Enophthalmos occurs because of oculosympathetic paresis [102]. (Redrawn and modified from Kanagalingam et al. [103])

2.4 Resistance to Thyroid Hormone

2.4.1 Goiter

Clinical Features
Goiter is quite frequent in patients with thyroid hormone resistance syndromes, a state of differential tissue insensitivity to circulating thyroid hormone, with a reported prevalence of 66–95% [105].

Pathophysiology
Impaired negative feedback inhibition of central thyrotropes in the setting of thyroid hormone resistance promotes TSH-mediated thyromegaly [106].

2.4.2 Short Stature

Clinical Features
In a prospective study at the National Institutes of Health, including 104 patients with thyroid hormone resistance, 18% had short stature [107].

Pathophysiology

- T3 acts on thyroid hormone receptors present on chondrocytes in the growth plate and plays a critical role in their differentiation and maturation [108]. Reduced levels of T3, as occurs in hypothyroidism, leads to thinning of both the proliferative and hypertrophic zones of the growth plate [109].
- T3 potentiates the local production of IGF-1 in the growth plate [108] (see Sect. 1.5.1). Hypothyroid subjects have impaired longitudinal growth due to the blunted effects of T3 on the GH-IGF1 axis [109].

 Pathophysiology Pearl

Thyroid hormone resistance

  Thyroid hormone resistance (THR) states occur as a result of mutations in the genes responsible for the various subtypes of the thyroid hormone receptor [105, 110, 111]. The thyroid hormone receptor alpha (THRA) and thyroid hormone receptor beta (THRB) genes code for TRα and TRβ subtypes of the thyroid hormone receptor, respectively [111–113].

  There is a variable expression of these receptors in different tissues, accounting for the lack of consistent clinical findings in patients with THR [113, 114].

  Pituitary or central thyroid hormone resistance occurs due to impaired negative feedback of the circulating thyroid hormone on the pituitary thyrotropes. Patients are usually clinically hyperthyroid [115]. In contrast, patients with generalized thyroid hormone resistance may be euthyroid, hypothyroid, or hyperthyroid, depending on the predominant tissue-specific thyroid hormone receptor subtype affected [112].

 Questions You Might Be Asked on Rounds

Does TSH hypersecretion due to thyroid hormone resistance lead to thyroid adenomas or cancer?

  TSH hypersecretion causes mild enlargement of the thyroid gland, but there is no evidence that it increases the risk of either adenoma or malignancy [116].

What is the eponymous name for thyroid hormone resistance syndromes?

  The first case of thyroid hormone resistance was described in 1967 by Dr. Samuel Refetoff and his colleagues [106]. "Refetoff syndrome" was first used in a published case report from Japan [117]. Subsequent case reports have since used this eponymous term [118–120].

2.5   Medullary Thyroid Cancer

2.5.1   Facial Flushing and Other Clinical Features of Neuroendocrine Origin

Clinical Features
Patients with medullary thyroid cancer can present with facial flushing. It is described as a "dry flush" due to the absence of associated cutaneous sweating [121], in contrast to the "wet flush" of menopause [122].

Pathophysiology
The parafollicular cells of the thyroid gland are derived from cells of neural crest origin, which have been aptly named APUD (amine precursor uptake decarboxylation) cells. These neuroendocrine cells can release various amines, including serotonin, histamine, prostaglandins, and ACTH [123]. Cutaneous flushing and diarrhea due to these amines are discussed in Sects. 4.4.1 and 4.4.2, respectively.

2.5.2   Cervical Mass

Clinical Features
The most frequent clinical finding in MTC is the presence of a mass or nodule in the cervical region, with a reported prevalence of 35% to 50%. Neck findings could be due to cervical lymph node involvement or compressive neck symptoms due to an enlarged thyroid nodule [124].

Pathophysiology
MTC occurs due to malignant transformation of parafollicular cells [125], which are of neural crest origin [124]. A mutation of the rearranged during transfection (RET) proto-oncogene results in the clonal proliferation of parafollicular cells [125].

 Questions You Might Be Asked on Rounds
Which endocrine conditions present with MTC? [126].

- Multiple endocrine neoplasia type 2A and 2B.
- Familial medullary thyroid carcinoma (FMTC).
- Sporadic MTC occurs much later in life between 40 and 60 years of age. Hereditary MTC encompasses MEN type 2 syndromes and FMTC and tends to occur much earlier in life compared to sporadic MTC [127].

At what age and in which specific inherited endocrinopathies should prophylactic total thyroidectomy be performed? [128].
Patients should have a total thyroidectomy by 5 years of age if they have MEN2A with germline mutation involving the RET codon at position 634 or MEN2B.

References

1. Lane Furdell E. Eponymous, anonymous: queen Anne's sign and the misnaming of a symptom. J Med Biogr. 2007;15:97–101.
2. Feingold KR, Elias PM. Endocrine-skin interactions. Cutaneous manifestations of pituitary disease, thyroid disease, calcium disorders, and diabetes. J Am Acad Dermatol. 1987;17:921–40.
3. van Beek N, Bodó E, Kromminga A, Gáspár E, Meyer K, Zmijewski MA, Slominski A, Wenzel BE, Paus R. Thyroid hormones directly Alter human hair follicle functions: Anagen prolongation and stimulation of both hair matrix keratinocyte proliferation and hair pigmentation. J Clin Endocrinol Metab. 2008;93:4381–8.
4. Parrino D, Di Bella S. Hertoghe sign: a hallmark of lepromatous leprosy. QJM Int J Med. 2016;109:497.
5. Kumar A, Karthikeyan K. Madarosis: a marker of Many maladies. Int J Trichology. 2012;4:3–18.
6. Ozcan KS, Osmonov D, Erdinler I, et al. Atrioventricular block in patients with thyroid dysfunction: prognosis after treatment with hormone supplementation or antithyroid medication. J Cardiol. 2012;60:327–32.
7. Dillmann W h. Cellular action of thyroid hormone on the heart. Thyroid. 2002;12:447–52.
8. Sun Z-Q, Ojamaa K, Nakamura TY, Artman M, Klein I, Coetzee WA. Thyroid hormone increases pacemaker activity in rat neonatal atrial Myocytes. J Mol Cell Cardiol. 2001;33:811–24.
9. Kabadi UM, Kumar SP. Pericardial effusion in primary hypothyroidism. Am Heart J. 1990;120:1393–5.
10. Apaydin M, Beysel S, Demirci T, Caliskan M, Kizilgul M, Ozcelik O, Cakal E, Delibasi T. A case of primary hypothyroidism initially presenting with massive pericardial effusion. J Clin Transl Endocrinol Case Rep. 2016;2:1–2.
11. Wong CL, Holroyd-Leduc J, Straus SE. Does this patient have a pleural effusion? JAMA. 2009;301:309–17.
12. Stolz L, Valenzuela J, Situ-LaCasse E, Stolz U, Hawbaker N, Thompson M, Adhikari S. Clinical and historical features of emergency department patients with pericardial effusions. World J Emerg Med. 2017;8:29–33.
13. Malahfji M, Arain S. Reversed Pulsus Paradoxus in right ventricular failure. Methodist Debakey Cardiovasc J. 2018;14:298–300.
14. Parving H-H, Hansen JM, Nielsen SL, Rossing N, Munck O, Lassen NA. Mechanisms of edema formation in myxedema — increased protein extravasation and relatively slow lymphatic drainage. N Engl J Med. 1979;301:460–5.
15. Rothschild MA, Bauman A, Yalow RS, Berson SA. Tissue distribution of I131 labeled human serum albumin following intravenous administration. J Clin Invest. 1955;34:1354–8.
16. Safer JD. Thyroid hormone action on skin. Dermatoendocrinol. 2011;3:211–5.
17. Keen MA, Hassan I, Bhat MH. A clinical study of the cutaneous manifestations of hypothyroidism in Kashmir Valley. Indian J Dermatol. 2013;58:326.
18. Indra R, Patil SS, Joshi R, Pai M, Kalantri SP. Accuracy of physical examination in the diagnosis of hypothyroidism: a cross-sectional, double-blind study. J Postgrad Med. 2004;50:7–11.
19. Heymann WR. Cutaneous manifestations of thyroid disease. J Am Acad Dermatol. 1992;26:885–902.
20. Ai J, Leonhardt JM, Heymann WR. Autoimmune thyroid diseases: etiology, pathogenesis, and dermatologic manifestations. J Am Acad Dermatol. 2003;48:641–62.
21. Loevy HT, Aduss H, Rosenthal IM. Tooth eruption and craniofacial development in congenital hypothyroidism: report of case. J Am Dent Assoc. 1987;115:429–31.
22. Murthy P, Laing MR. Macroglossia. BMJ. 1994;309:1386–7.
23. Melville JC, Menegotto KD, Woernley TC, Maida BD, Alava I. Unusual case of a massive Macroglossia secondary to myxedema: a case report and literature review. J Oral Maxillofac Surg. 2018;76:119–27.

24. Sosnay PR, Kim S. Images in clinical medicine. Hypothyroid-induced hyporeflexia N Engl J Med. 2006;354:e27.
25. Burkholder DB, Klaas JP, Kumar N, Boes CJ. The origin of Woltman's sign of myxoedema. J Clin Neurosci. 2013;20:1204–6.
26. Houston CS. The diagnostic importance of the myxoedema reflex (Woltman's sign). Can Med Assoc J. 1958;78:108–12.
27. Krishnamurthy A, Vishnu VY, Hamide A. Clinical signs in hypothyroidism—myoedema and Woltman sign. QJM Int J Med. 2018;111:193.
28. Bloise FF, Cordeiro A, Ortiga-Carvalho TM. Role of thyroid hormone in skeletal muscle physiology. J Endocrinol. 2018;236:R57–68.
29. Madariaga MG. Polymyositis-like syndrome in hypothyroidism: review of cases reported over the past twenty-five years. Thyroid Off J Am Thyroid Assoc. 2002;12:331–6.
30. Duyff RF, Van den Bosch J, Laman DM, van Loon BJ, Linssen WH. Neuromuscular findings in thyroid dysfunction: a prospective clinical and electrodiagnostic study. J Neurol Neurosurg Psychiatry. 2000;68:750–5.
31. Klein I, Parker M, Shebert R, Ayyar DR, Levey GS. Hypothyroidism presenting as muscle stiffness and pseudohypertrophy: Hoffmann's syndrome. Am J Med. 1981;70:891–4.
32. Mangaraj S, Sethy G. Hoffman's syndrome – a rare facet of hypothyroid myopathy. J Neurosci Rural Pract. 2014;5:447–8.
33. Salvatore D, Simonides WS, Dentice M, Zavacki AM, Larsen PR. Thyroid hormones and skeletal muscle — new insights and potential implications. Nat Rev Endocrinol. 2014;10:206–14.
34. Honbo KS, van Herle AJ, Kellett KA. Serum prolactin levels in untreated primary hypothyroidism. Am J Med. 1978;64:782–7.
35. Ansari MS, Almalki MH. Primary hypothyroidism with markedly high prolactin. Front Endocrinol. 2016; https://doi.org/10.3389/fendo.2016.00035.
36. Johnston PC, Ellis PK, Hunter SJ. Thyrotroph hyperplasia. Postgrad Med J. 2014;90:56–7.
37. Kocova M, Netkov S, Sukarova-Angelovska E. Pituitary Pseudotumor with unusual presentation reversed shortly after the introduction of Thyroxine replacement therapy. J Pediatr Endocrinol Metab. 2011;14:1665–70.
38. Shahbaz A, Aziz K, Umair M, Sachmechi I. Prolonged duration of Hashitoxicosis in a patient with Hashimoto's thyroiditis: a case report and review of literature. Cureus. 2018;10:e2804.
39. Gillespie EF, Smith TJ, Douglas RS. Thyroid eye disease: towards an evidence base for treatment in the 21st century. Curr Neurol Neurosci Rep. 2012;12:318–24.
40. Bahn RS. Graves' Ophthalmopathy. N Engl J Med. 2010;362:726–38.
41. McAlinden C. An overview of thyroid eye disease. Eye Vis. 2014;1:9.
42. Gupta S, Douglas R. The pathophysiology of thyroid eye disease (TED): implications for immunotherapy. Curr Opin Ophthalmol. 2011;22:385–90.
43. Douglas RS, Kahaly GJ, Patel A, et al. Teprotumumab for the treatment of active thyroid eye disease. N Engl J Med. 2020;382:341–52.
44. Smith TJ. Potential role for bone marrow-derived fibrocytes in the orbital fibroblast heterogeneity associated with thyroid-associated ophthalmopathy. Clin Exp Immunol. 2010;162:24–31.
45. Mallika P, Tan A, Aziz S, Alwi SS, Chong M, Vanitha R, Intan G. Thyroid associated Ophthalmopathy – a review. Malays Fam Physician Off J Acad Fam Physicians Malays. 2009;4:8–14.
46. Urrets-Zavalía JA, Espósito E, Garay I, Monti R, Ruiz-Lascano A, Correa L, Serra HM, Grzybowski A. The eye and the skin in endocrine metabolic diseases. Clin Dermatol. 2016;34:151–65.
47. Khatavi F, Nasrollahi K, Zandi A, Panahi M, Mortazavi M, Pourazizi M, Ranjbar-Omidi B. A promising modified procedure for upper eyelid retraction-associated graves' Ophthalmopathy: Transconjunctival lateral Levator Aponeurectomy. Med Hypothesis Discov Innov Ophthalmol. 2017;6:44–8.
48. Bartley GB. The differential diagnosis and classification of eyelid retraction. Trans Am Ophthalmol Soc. 1995;93:371–89.

49. Kishimoto I, Chuyen NTH, Okamoto H. Annularly arranged nodular pretibial myxedema after 7-year treatment of graves' disease. J Dermatol. 2018;45:110–1.
50. Sendhil Kumaran M, Dutta P, Sakia U, Dogra S. Long-term follow-up and epidemiological trends in patients with pretibial myxedema: an 11-year study from a tertiary care center in northern India. Int J Dermatol. 2015;54:e280–6.
51. di Meo N, Nan K, Noal C, Trevisini S, Fadel M, Damiani G, Vichi S, Trevisan G. Polypoid and fungating form of elephantiasic pretibial myxedema with involvement of the hands. Int J Dermatol. 2016;55:e413–5.
52. Chang TC, Kao SC, Huang KM. Octreotide and graves' ophthalmopathy and pretibial myxoedema. BMJ. 1992;304:158.
53. Girgis CM, Champion BL, Wall JR. Current concepts in graves' disease. Ther Adv Endocrinol Metab. 2011;2:135–44.
54. Jabbour SA. Cutaneous manifestations of endocrine disorders: a guide for dermatologists. Am J Clin Dermatol. 2003;4:315–31.
55. Serrao R, Zirwas M, English JC. Palmar erythema. Am J Clin Dermatol. 2007;8:347–56.
56. Ruggeri RM, Imbesi S, Saitta S, Campennì A, Cannavò S, Trimarchi F, Gangemi S. Chronic idiopathic urticaria and graves' disease. J Endocrinol Investig. 2013;36:531–6.
57. Casadio R, Santi V, Mirici-Cappa F, Magini G, Cacciari M, Bernardi M, Trevisani F. Telangiectasia as a presenting sign of graves' disease. Horm Res. 2008;69:189–92.
58. Gul M, Katz J, Chaudhry AA, Hannah-Shmouni F, Skarulis M, Cochran CS. Rheumatologic and imaging manifestations of thyroid Acropachy. Arthritis Rheumatol. 2016;68:1636.
59. Fatourechi V. Thyroid dermopathy and acropachy. Best Pract Res Clin Endocrinol Metab. 2012;26:553–65.
60. Fatourechi V, Ahmed DDF, Schwartz KM. Thyroid Acropachy: report of 40 patients treated at a single institution in a 26-year period. J Clin Endocrinol Metab. 2002;87:5435–41.
61. Luria MN, Asper SPJR. Onycholysis in hyperthyroidism. Ann Intern Med. 1958;49:102–8.
62. Atia A, Johnson B, Abdelmalak H, Sinnott B. Visual Vignette. Endocr Pract. 2008;14:132.
63. Ghayee HK, Mattern JQA, Cooper DS. Dirty nails. J Clin Endocrinol Metab. 2005;90:2428.
64. Joshi KK, de Bock M, Choong CC. Graves' disease presenting as life-threatening hypokalaemic periodic paralysis. J Paediatr Child Health. 2017;54:443–5.
65. Falhammar H, Thorén M, Calissendorff J. Thyrotoxic periodic paralysis: clinical and molecular aspects. Endocrine. 2013;43:274–84.
66. Sonkar SK, Kumar S, Singh NK. Thyrotoxic hypokalemic periodic paralysis. Indian J Crit Care Med. 2018;22:378.
67. Rhee EP, Scott JA, Dighe AS. Case records of the Massachusetts General Hospital. Case 4-2012. A 37-year-old man with muscle pain, weakness, and weight loss. N Engl J Med. 2012;366:553–60.
68. Williams E, Chillag S, Rizvi A. Thyroid Bruit and the Underlying 'Inferno. Am J Med. 2014;127:489–90.
69. Rich K. Carotid bruit: A review. J Vasc Nurs. 2015;33:26–7.
70. Bindra A, Braunstein GD. Thyroiditis. Am Fam Physician. 2006;73:1769–76.
71. Panagoulis C, Halapas A, Chariatis E, Driva P, Matsakas E. Hyperthyroidism and the heart. Hell J Cardiol HJC Hell Kardiologike Epitheorese. 2008;49:169–75.
72. Taggar JS, Coleman T, Lewis S, Heneghan C, Jones M. Accuracy of methods for detecting an irregular pulse and suspected atrial fibrillation: a systematic review and meta-analysis. Eur J Prev Cardiol. 2016;23:1330–8.
73. Ertek S, Cicero AF. Hyperthyroidism and cardiovascular complications: a narrative review on the basis of pathophysiology. Arch Med Sci AMS. 2013;9:944–52.
74. Almeida NAS, Cordeiro A, Machado DS, Souza LL, Ortiga-Carvalho TM, Campos-de-Carvalho AC, Wondisford FE, Pazos-Moura CC. Connexin40 messenger ribonucleic acid is positively regulated by thyroid hormone (TH) acting in cardiac atria via the TH receptor. Endocrinology. 2009;150:546–54.

75. Cacciatori V, Bellavere F, Pezzarossa A, Dellera A, Gemma ML, Thomaseth K, Castello R, Moghetti P, Muggeo M. Power spectral analysis of heart rate in hyperthyroidism. J Clin Endocrinol Metab. 1996;81:2828–35.
76. Chan WB, Yeung VTF, Chow CC, So WY, Cockram CS. Gynaecomastia as a presenting feature of thyrotoxicosis. Postgrad Med J. 1999;75:229–31.
77. Kumar KVSH, Kumar A, Bansal R, Kalia R. Bilateral gynecomastia: a rare presentation of thyrotoxicosis. Indian J Endocrinol Metab. 2013;17:357–8.
78. Choong K, Safer J. Graves disease and gynecomastia in 2 roommates. Endocr Pract. 2011;17:647–50.
79. Ohta T, Nishioka M, Nakata N, Fukuda K, Shirakawa T. Significance of perithyroidal lymph nodes in benign thyroid diseases. J Med Ultrason. 2018;45:81–7.
80. Hadjkacem F, Ghorbel D, Mnif F, Elfekih H, Rekik N, Mrabet H, Ammar M, Charfi N, Abid M. Lymphoid hyperplasia in graves. 2017; https://doi.org/10.1530/endoabs.49.EP1349.
81. Kim MJ, Cho SW, Choi S, Ju DL, Park DJ, Park YJ. Changes in body compositions and basal metabolic rates during treatment of graves' disease. Int J Endocrinol. 2018; https://doi.org/10.1155/2018/9863050.
82. Porter C. Quantification of UCP1 function in human brown adipose tissue. Adipocytes. 2017;6:167–74.
83. Carvalho DP, Dupuy C. Thyroid hormone biosynthesis and release. Mol Cell Endocrinol. 2017;458:6–15.
84. Takasu N, Nakachi K, Higa H. Development of graves' hyperthyroidism caused an adrenal crisis in a patient with previously unrecognized non-classical 21-hydroxylase deficiency. Intern Med Tokyo Jpn. 2010;49:1395–400.
85. Daumerie C, Ludgate M, Costagliola S, Many MC. Evidence for thyrotropin receptor immunoreactivity in pretibial connective tissue from patients with thyroid-associated dermopathy. Eur J Endocrinol. 2002;146:35–8.
86. Pemberton HS. Sign of submerged goitre. Lancet. 1946;248:509.
87. De Filippis EA, Sabet A, Sun MRM, Garber JR. Pemberton's sign: explained nearly 70 years later. J Clin Endocrinol Metab. 2014;99:1949–54.
88. Katoh H, Enomoto T, Watanabe M. Superior vena cava syndrome due to mediastinal adenomatous goitre. BMJ Case Rep. 2015;2015:bcr2015210634.
89. Cakir E. Superior vena cava syndrome due to enlarged thyroid gland. 2013; https://doi.org/10.1530/endoabs.32.P1063.
90. Marcelino M, Nobre E, Conceição J, Lopes L, Vilar H, de Castro JJ. Superior vena cava syndrome and substernal goiter. Thyroid. 2010;20:235–6.
91. Manning PB, Thompson NW. Bilateral phrenic nerve palsy associated with benign thyroid goiter. Acta Chir Scand. 1989;155:429–31.
92. van Doorn LG, Kranendonk SE. Partial unilateral phrenic nerve paralysis caused by a large intrathoracic goitre. Neth J Med. 1996;48:216–9.
93. Benbakh M, Abou-elfadl M, Rouadi S, Abada R-L, Roubal M, Mahtar M. Substernal goiter: experience with 50 cases. Eur Ann Otorhinolaryngol Head Neck Dis. 2016;133:19–22.
94. Hakeem AH, Hakeem IH, Wani FJ. Phrenic nerve palsy as initial presentation of large retrosternal goitre. Indian J Surg Oncol. 2016;7:460–3.
95. Jiang S, Xu W-D, Shen Y-D, Xu J-G, Gu Y-D. An anatomical study of the full-length phrenic nerve and its blood supply: clinical implications for endoscopic dissection. Anat Sci Int. 2011;86:225–31.
96. Lewinski A. The problem of goitre with particular consideration of goitre resulting from iodine deficiency (I): classification, diagnostics and treatment. Neuro Endocrinol Lett. 2002;23:351–5.
97. Abuye C, Berhane Y, Akalu G, Getahun Z, Ersumo T. Prevalence of goiter in children 6 to 12 years of age in Ethiopia. Food Nutr Bull. 2007;28:391–8.
98. Paschke R. Molecular pathogenesis of nodular goiter. Langenbeck's Arch Surg. 2011;396:1127–36.

99. Falhammar H, Juhlin CC, Barner C, Catrina S-B, Karefylakis C, Calissendorff J. Riedel's thyroiditis: clinical presentation, treatment and outcomes. Endocrine. 2018;60:185–92.
100. Dahlgren M, Khosroshahi A, Nielsen GP, Deshpande V, Stone JH. Riedel's thyroiditis and multifocal Fibrosclerosis are part of the IgG4-related systemic disease spectrum. Arthritis Care Res. 2010;62:1312–8.
101. Soh S-B, Pham A, O'Hehir RE, Cherk M, Topliss DJ. Novel use of rituximab in a case of Riedel's thyroiditis refractory to glucocorticoids and Tamoxifen. J Clin Endocrinol Metab. 2013;98:3543–9.
102. Amonoo-Kuofi HS. Horner's syndrome revisited: with an update of the central pathway. Clin Anat N Y N. 1999;12:345–61.
103. Kanagalingam S, Miller NR. Horner syndrome: clinical perspectives. Eye Brain. 2015;7:35–46.
104. Leuchter I, Becker M, Mickel R, Dulguerov P. Horner's syndrome and thyroid neoplasms. ORL J Oto-Rhino-Laryngol Its Relat Spec. 2002;64:49–52.
105. Weiss RE, Dumitrescu A, Refetoff S. Approach to the patient with resistance to thyroid hormone and pregnancy. J Clin Endocrinol Metab. 2010;95:3094–102.
106. Refetoff S, Dewind LT, Degroot LJ. Familial syndrome combining deaf-Mutism, stippled epiphyses, goiter and abnormally high PBI: possible target organ refractoriness to thyroid hormone. J Clin Endocrinol Metab. 1967;27:279–94.
107. Brucker-Davis F, Skarulis MC, Grace MB, Benichou J, Hauser P, Wiggs E, Weintraub BD. Genetic and clinical features of 42 kindreds with resistance to thyroid hormone. The National Institutes of Health prospective study. Ann Intern Med. 1995;123:572–83.
108. Kim H-Y, Mohan S. Role and mechanisms of actions of thyroid hormone on the skeletal development. Bone Res. 2013;1:146–61.
109. Nilsson O, Marino R, De Luca F, Phillip M, Baron J. Endocrine regulation of the growth plate. Horm Res. 2005;64:157–65.
110. Tylki-Szymańska A, Acuna-Hidalgo R, Krajewska-Walasek M, et al. Thyroid hormone resistance syndrome due to mutations in the thyroid hormone receptor α gene (THRA). J Med Genet. 2015;52:312–6.
111. Rivas AM, Lado-Abeal J. Thyroid hormone resistance and its management. Proc Bayl Univ Med Cent. 2016;29:209–11.
112. Moran C, Chatterjee K. Resistance to thyroid hormone due to defective thyroid receptor alpha. Best Pract Res Clin Endocrinol Metab. 2015;29:647–57.
113. Moran C, Agostini M, Visser WE, et al. Resistance to thyroid hormone due to a mutation in thyroid hormone receptor α1 and the α2 variant protein. Lancet Diabetes Endocrinol. 2014;2:619–26.
114. Lee JH, Kim EY. Resistance to thyroid hormone due to a novel mutation of thyroid hormone receptor beta gene. Ann Pediatr Endocrinol Metab. 2014;19:229–31.
115. Agrawal NK, Goyal R, Rastogi A, Naik D, Singh SK. Thyroid hormone resistance. Postgrad Med J. 2008;84:473–7.
116. Weiss RE, Refetoff S. Treatment of resistance to thyroid hormone—Primum non Nocere. J Clin Endocrinol Metab. 1999;84:401–4.
117. Yamada K, Takamatsu J, Takeda K, Sakane S, Hishitani Y. Generalized resistance to thyroid hormone (Refetoff syndrome) associated with abnormal secretion of growth hormone and prolactin: a case report. Nihon Naika Gakkai Zasshi J Jpn Soc Intern Med. 1988;77:1556–60.
118. Inada S, Iwasaki Y, Tugita M, Hashimoto K. Thyroid hormone resistance (Refetoff syndrome) incidentally found in a patient with primary hyperparathyroidism. Nihon Naika Gakkai Zasshi J Jpn Soc Intern Med. 2007;96:1706–8.
119. Sambalingam D, Rao KJ. Neonatal "resistance to thyroid hormone (refetoff syndrome)" with novel THRB mutation. J Clin Neonatol. 2017;6:273.
120. Alberto G, Novi RF, Scalabrino E, Trombetta A, Seardo MA, Maurino M, Brossa C. Atrial fibrillation and mitral prolapse in a subject affected by Refetoff syndrome. Minerva Cardioangiol. 2002;50:157–60.

121. Rastogi V, Singh D, Mazza JJ, Parajuli D, Yale SH. Flushing disorders associated with gastro-intestinal symptoms: part 1, neuroendocrine tumors, mast cell disorders and Hyperbasophila. Clin Med Res. 2018;16:16–28.
122. Sturdee DW, Hunter MS, Maki PM, Gupta P, Sassarini J, Stevenson JC, Lumsden MA. The menopausal hot flush: a review. Climacteric. 2017;20:296–305.
123. Cai S, Deng H, Chen Y, Wu X, Guan X. Treatment of medullary thyroid carcinoma with apatinib: a case report and literature review. Medicine (Baltimore). 2017;96:e8704.
124. Roy M, Chen H, Sippel RS. Current understanding and Management of Medullary Thyroid Cancer. Oncologist. 2013;18:1093–100.
125. Lin S-F, Lin J-D, Hsueh C, Chou T-C, Wong RJ. Activity of roniciclib in medullary thyroid cancer. Oncotarget. 2018;9:28030–41.
126. A T, F S, G P, M B. Genetic alterations in medullary thyroid Cancer: diagnostic and prognostic markers. Curr Genomics. 2011;12:618–25.
127. Wells SA, Asa SL, Dralle H, et al. Revised American Thyroid Association guidelines for the management of medullary thyroid carcinoma. Thyroid Off J Am Thyroid Assoc. 2015;25:567–610.
128. American Thyroid Association Guidelines Task Force, Kloos RT, Eng C, et al. Medullary thyroid cancer: management guidelines of the American Thyroid Association. Thyroid Off J Am Thyroid Assoc. 2009;19:565–612.

Adrenal Gland Signs

3

Learning Objectives
At the end of this chapter, you will be able to:

1. Understand the renin-angiotensin-aldosterone (RAA) axis and the factors involved in both positive and negative feedback regulation
2. Appreciate the target effects of aldosterone and how perturbations in the RAA hormonal milieu result in specific clinical signs
3. Understand the role of cortisol in catecholamine metabolism
4. Understand the cardiovascular effects of catecholamines
5. Recognize the genetic basis for glucocorticoid-resistant states and appreciate the pathophysiologic basis of their clinical manifestations

3.1 Primary Adrenal Insufficiency

3.1.1 Postural Hypotension

Clinical Features
Arterial blood pressure decreases in patients with primary adrenocortical insufficiency [1]. Orthostatic hypotension can be elicited at the bedside by confirming a postural drop in blood pressure in changing from a supine to a semi-recumbent position or standing position [2].

Pathophysiology
1. Autoimmune-mediated destruction of the adrenal cortex results in reduced production of mineralocorticoids needed to maintain sodium and water balance [3] (see Fig. 3.1).

© Springer Nature Switzerland AG 2020
A. Manni, A. Quarde, *Endocrine Pathophysiology*,
https://doi.org/10.1007/978-3-030-49872-6_3

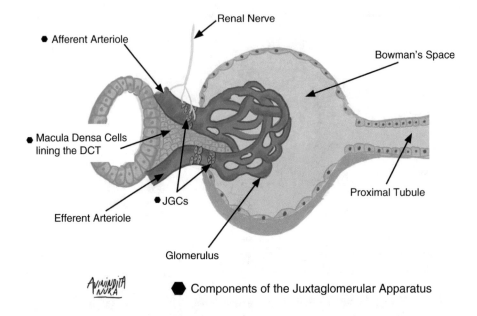

Fig. 3.1 The components of the juxtaglomerular apparatus. Triggers of renin secretion include a low sodium load presented to macula densa cells (located in the DCT), adrenergic stimulation from renal nerves innervating JGCs in the afferent arteriole, and a reduced tensile stretch of the afferent arteriole of the glomerulus. Renin, the rate-limiting enzyme in the renin-angiotensin-aldosterone system (RAAS), is critical in maintaining intravascular volume and blood pressure [7]. Renin release is also controlled by long and short negative feedback loops mediated by the effect of ATII on the collecting tubule and JGCs, respectively [9]. (Redrawn and modified from Alessandro et al. [9])

2. There is a single study to date, exploring the role of adrenomedullin in Addison's disease. Adrenomedullin (AM), a novel hypotensive peptide, was found to be high in patients with proven Addison's disease. There was, however, a weak correlation (r = 0.458; P value = 0.048) between systolic blood pressure and plasma AM levels in subjects with adrenocortical insufficiency. The authors were unable to explain the exact mechanism accounting for the high levels of AM in patients with Addison's disease [4].
3. Cortisol is critical in maintaining vascular tone through several mechanisms. Glucocorticoids potentiate the vasoconstrictive effect of catecholamines on vascular α1-receptors. An increase in vascular adrenergic receptor density is induced by glucocorticoids [5].
4. Similar to the effects of glucocorticoids on adrenergic receptors, vascular receptors of angiotensin II are upregulated by glucocorticoids [5].
5. Glucocorticoids increase the transcription of angiotensinogen, a precursor of angiotensin II [5].

Pathophysiology Pearl

Mechanisms of Renin Release

The juxtaglomerular apparatus is composed of the macula densa cells present in the distal convoluted tubule (DCT), juxtaglomerular cells (present in the entire glomerular vasculature but more prominent in the afferent arteriole), and the glomerular afferent arteriole (AT) [6]. See Fig. 3.1.

Renin, an enzyme released from *juxtaglomerular cells*, initiates a cascade of reactions, which leads to the eventual formation of angiotensin II (ATII) [7].

- Change in sodium chloride load presented to the macula densa cells (a group of 15–20 cells in the distal convoluted tubule) influences the eventual release of renin from the juxtaglomerular cells (JGCs), through some signaling mediators. A high sodium load inhibits renin release from the juxtaglomerular cells, whereas a low sodium load does the opposite [8].
- A change in blood pressure at the afferent arteriole controls renin release from the JGCs. Low tension in the afferent arteriolar wall increases renin release, which ultimately enhances sodium conservation and maintenance of intravascular volume [8].
- Activation of beta-adrenergic sympathetic nerves terminating in the juxtaglomerular cells promotes renin release [8].

Clinical Pearl

Biochemical Monitoring of Mineralocorticoid Replacement Therapy

Management of patients with primary adrenal insufficiency requires monitoring of mineralocorticoid replacement therapy to prevent hypertension, edema, and hypokalemia. The goal is to maintain plasma renin activity close to the upper limit of normal [10].

3.1.2 Hyperpigmentation

Clinical Features

Addison's disease presents with a classic dermatologic feature of hyperpigmentation involving sun-exposed areas, areas of prior trauma, palmar creases, oral mucosa, conjunctivae, and the nails (dark longitudinal ridges referred to as melanonychia) [11].

Pathophysiology

1. Melanogenesis is induced by α-melanocyte-stimulating hormone (MSH) acting on type 1 melanocortin receptors (MC1-R), present on melanocytes [12].
2. ACTH also binds to MC1-R receptors present on melanocytes [12]. Elevated levels of ACTH, as occurs in Addison's disease, contribute to hyperpigmentation of the skin.
3. Interestingly, all POMC-derived peptides have receptors on melanocytes, fibroblasts, and keratinocytes [12].

☀ **Pathophysiology Pearl**

Mediators of Melanin Formation (Fig. 3.2)

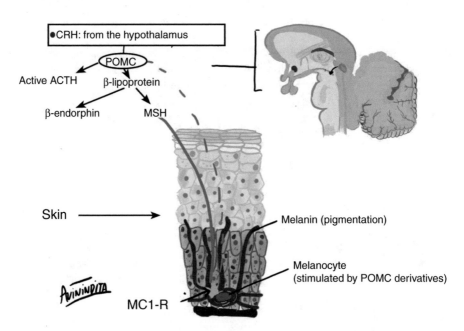

Fig. 3.2 Melanogenesis – the role of POMC derivatives in melanocyte activation. Corticotropin-releasing hormone (CRH) from the hypothalamus has a stimulating effect on the production of proopiomelanocortin (POMC) and its downstream products in the anterior pituitary gland. Adrenocorticotrophic hormone (ACTH) and beta-lipotropin are derived from POMC. Beta-lipotropin is subsequently cleaved to form beta-endorphin and melanocyte-stimulating hormone (MSH). MSH binds its cognate melanocyte 1 receptor (MC1-R) on the melanocyte to activate melanogenesis (solid line). Also, both POMC and ACTH can bind the MC1-R receptor and augment melanin production (dashed line) [12]. (Based on Yamamoto et al [12])

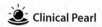 **Clinical Pearl**

The Houssay Phenomenon

Houssay phenomenon is an eponymous termed named after the Nobel Prize Laureate Dr. Bernardo Houssay. It is defined as significant hypoglycemia due to cortisol deficiency in the setting of panhypopituitarism. Patients with pre-existing diabetes may experience either resolution of diabetes or new-onset recurrent hypoglycemia due to the loss of the metabolic effects of crucial counterregulatory glucocorticoids [13].

 Questions on Clinical Rounds

What about the vascular supply of the adrenal gland that predisposes it to hemorrhage in the setting of coagulopathy?

Each adrenal gland is drained by a single adrenal vein, which makes it susceptible to veno-occlusive disease in the setting of coagulopathy. The left adrenal vein forms a confluence with the inferior phrenic vein and finally drains into the left renal vein. The right adrenal vein, however, drains directly into the inferior vena cava [14, 15].

What are the other clinical features of Addison's disease (Table 3.1)?

3.2   Primary Hyperaldosteronism

3.2.1 Hypertension

Clinical Features

Primary hyperaldosteronism happens to be the most common cause of secondary hypertension, with a reported prevalence of 5–10% among all hypertensive patients and as high as 20% in those with resistant hypertension [19].

Table 3.1 Clinical features grouped by the underlying mechanism

Clinical features	Underlying mechanism
Postural dizziness, hypotension, salt craving, and weight loss	Mineralocorticoid insufficiency [16]
Confusion, pallor, and diaphoresis	Hypocortisolemia-induced hypoglycemia [16]
Nausea, vomiting, and abdominal discomfort	The pathophysiology is uncertain [17]
Loss of androgen-dependent hair (adolescents, females) and reduced libido	Androgen deficiency [18]
Vitiligo	Autoimmune-mediated destruction of melanocytes [18]

Adapted from Park [16] Mandadi [17] and Auron [18]

Pathophysiology

Aldosterone promotes nuclear transcription and translation of the amiloride-sensitive epithelial sodium channels, which increases sodium and water conservation (see Fig. 3.3) [20].

There are mineralocorticoid receptors on vascular endothelial cells. Aldosterone plays an active role in both vasoconstriction and vasodilation; the circumstances under which it performs these roles are, however, yet to be elucidated [20]. Nonetheless, aldosterone excess induces mineralocorticoid receptor overactivation, inflammation of the vascular endothelium, and myocardial remodeling, which are all critical contributory factors to the development of hypertension [20].

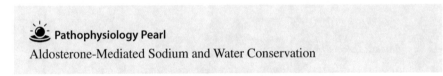

Pathophysiology Pearl

Aldosterone-Mediated Sodium and Water Conservation

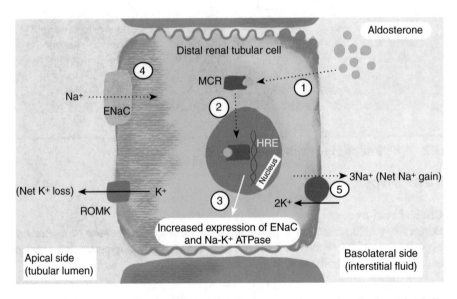

Fig. 3.3 Aldosterone-mediated sodium and water conservation at the distal renal tubule. Aldosterone, a lipid-soluble steroid hormone, diffuses through the cell membrane of the ductal epithelial cell and binds to the cytosolic mineralocorticoid receptor (MCR) (step 1). The aldosterone-MCR complex is then translocated into the nucleus where it attaches to the hormone response element (HRE) (step 2) required for transcription and translation of the epithelial sodium chloride (ENaC) channel and sodium-potassium adenosine triphosphatase (Na-K+ ATPase) pump (step 3). ENaC and Na-K+ ATPase both play an active role in sodium reabsorption from the filtered renal sodium load present in the collecting duct and distal convoluted tubule. The net effect is the transfer of sodium from the apical to the basolateral side of the renal tubular cell (steps 4 and 5) [19, 20]. Aldosterone also promotes the expression of renal outer medullary potassium (ROMK) channels. The insertion of ROMK channels on the apical membrane facilitates potassium and hydrogen ion loss [21]. (Redrawn and modified from Byrd et al. [19])

3.2.2 Muscle Weakness

Clinical Features

Significant muscle weakness can occur in patients with primary hyperaldosteronism. There are a few case reports of myopathy as the presenting feature of Conn's syndrome [22–24].

Pathophysiology

Aldosterone plays an active role in the upregulation of potassium (K^+) channels present on the apical surface of the ductal cell. These K^+ channels are involved in the extrusion of K^+ from the ductal cell into the lumen of the renal tubule (see Fig. 3.3). This accounts for the hypokalemia-induced muscle weakness seen in patients with primary hyperaldosteronism (see Fig. 3.3) [20].

3.2.3 Atrial Fibrillation

Clinical Features

An association of atrial fibrillation with hyperaldosteronism is widely accepted; there is, however, a paucity of prospective study data on the prevalence of atrial fibrillation in subjects with hyperaldosteronism [25]. Patients with primary aldosteronism are at a 12-fold risk of developing atrial fibrillation compared to patients with essential hypertension [26]. An irregularly irregular pulse rate and rhythm is the classic clinical finding in atrial fibrillation [27].

Pathophysiology

1. Mineralocorticoid receptors present on cardiac myocytes are activated by excess aldosterone, which results in myocyte hypertrophy. Left ventricular hypertrophy causes significant diastolic dysfunction and predisposes patients to atrial fibrillation [25].
2. Mineralocorticoid-mediated inflammation induces fibrosis of the myocardium. Multiple foci of fibrosis induce re-entry circuits in the heart, which increases the risk of atrial fibrillation [25].
3. Hyperaldosteronism-induced hypokalemia causes prolongation of the PR interval (extends the period of ventricular diastolic filling), which impairs diastolic function and, as mentioned in (1) above, predisposes the myocardium to arrhythmias [25].

3.2.4 Dehydration

Clinical Features

Patients with primary hyperaldosteronism can present with hypotonic polyuria and polydipsia [28].

Pathophysiology
Hyperaldosteronism increases potassium wasting at the distal renal tubules [28]. Hypokalemia subsequently promotes a downregulation of aquaporin-2 (AQP-2) channels on both cortical and inner medullary ductal cells, which results in renal free water loss [29].

Hypokalemia reduces intracellular cyclic adenosine monophosphate (cAMP) activity, a critical second messenger that mediates the effects of antidiuretic hormone (ADH) at the ductal cell. ADH is, therefore, unable to promote the insertion of AQP-2 water channels on the renal tubular apical membrane. This results in an acquired form of nephrogenic diabetes insipidus (see also Fig. 1.6) [28].

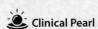 Clinical Pearl

Screening for Hyperaldosteronism

1. Hypokalemia inhibits aldosterone production; as such, potassium levels should be maintained at a level ≥ 4 mmol/L before screening for hyperaldosteronism with the aldosterone to renin ratio (ARR) [19].
2. Medications that interfere with ARR testing, such as mineralocorticoid antagonists and angiotensin-converting enzyme (ACE) inhibitors, may not need to be held before initial hyperaldosteronism screening. Indeed, if renin is suppressed in the setting of mineralocorticoid antagonist or ACE inhibitor therapy, then the ARR is interpretable. It is essential to bear this caveat in mind since the discontinuation of antihypertensives comes with risks such as poorly controlled hypertension or, worse still, hypertensive crises [19].

 Pathophysiology Pearl

Why do patients with primary hyperaldosteronism seldom develop peripheral edema despite the sodium and water-conserving effects of excess aldosterone?

1. An increase in sodium and water conservation elevates the cardiac preload and leads to stretching of the atrial cardiomyocytes. Atrial natriuretic factor is then released by the atrial cardiomyocytes, which promotes natriuresis (renal sodium loss) in the medullary collecting ducts of the nephron [30].
2. Increased renal perfusion pressures due to plasma volume expansion leads to "pressure natriuresis." The proximal tubule is unable to reabsorb enough sodium due to an increased filtered load in the setting of increased intraglomerular filtration pressures. This results in the delivery of a high renal tubular sodium load to the distal nephrons, which subsequently overwhelms the sodium-conserving effects of aldosterone (see Fig. 3.3) [30].

Questions You Might Be Asked on Clinical Rounds

What clinical features should prompt a clinician to screen a patient for primary hyperaldosteronism (Table 3.2)?

What are the causes of pseudohyperaldosteronism?

These are endocrine conditions that present with some of the clinical features of primary hyperaldosteronism (hypertension and hypokalemia) but do not exhibit the expected increase in plasma aldosterone to plasma renin ratio. Patients with pseudohyperaldosteronism have low levels of both aldosterone and renin [32] (Table 3.3).

Table 3.2 Screening recommendations for hyperaldosteronism

Endocrine Society screening recommendations:
Blood pressure above 150/100 mmHg; should be measured on three occasions on separate days [31]
Uncontrolled blood pressure on three or more antihypertensives, including a diuretic Δ [31]
Controlled blood pressure requiring four or more antihypertensive agents Δ [31]
Hypertension in the setting of sleep apnea or adrenal incidentaloma [31]
Hypertension with a family history of early-onset hypertension or stroke at <40 years of age [31]
First-degree hypertensive relatives of patients with primary hyperaldosteronism [31]

Δ Suggestive of resistant hypertension
Adapted from Funder et al. [31]

Table 3.3 Mechanisms underlying the various causes of pseudohyperaldosteronism

Condition	Mechanism
Liddle's syndrome	A gain-of-function mutation of the gene encoding the amiloride-sensitive epithelial sodium chloride transporter [33]
Gordon syndrome	A gain-of-function mutation of the thiazide-sensitive sodium chloride cotransporter in the distal nephron. Unlike other causes of pseudohyperaldosteronism, Gordon syndrome is associated with hyperkalemia instead of hypokalemia [34]
Defects in adrenal steroidogenesis	Deficiency of 11beta-hydroxylase enzyme results in a buildup of 11-deoxycorticosterone (which has intrinsic mineralocorticoid activity) [35]
Cushing's syndrome	Excess cortisol binds to the mineralocorticoid receptor due to saturation of the 11beta-hydroxysteroid dehydrogenase 2 enzyme (see the cortisol-to-cortisone shunt, Section 1.1.1) [36]
Apparent mineralocorticoid excess	An autosomal recessive condition characterized by an inactivating mutation of the 11beta-hydroxysteroid dehydrogenase 2 enzyme (see the cortisol-to-cortisone shunt, Section 1.1.1) [37]
Excessive intake of licorice, grapefruits, or carbenoxolone	Inhibition of 11beta-hydroxysteroid dehydrogenase 2 (see the cortisol-to-cortisone shunt, Section 1.1.1) [36]
Medication-induced	Corticosteroids and contraceptives [36]

Adapted from references [33–37]

3.3   Pseudohypoaldosteronism

3.3.1   Cardiac Arrest due to Life-Threatening Hyperkalemia

Clinical Features
Infants born with this condition present with sudden cardiac death [38, 39].

Pathophysiology
Pseudohypoaldosteronism type 1 (PHA1) can be inherited in either an autosomal dominant or recessive pattern. Loss-of-function mutations in either the mineralocorticoid receptor (MCR) or the amiloride-sensitive epithelial sodium chloride channel (ENaC) gene reduce the target organ effects of aldosterone. Refractory hyperkalemia can lead to peaked T waves, wide QRS complex, eventual ventricular arrhythmia, and asystole [38, 39]. Impaired action of aldosterone results in not only hyperkalemia but hyponatremia and metabolic acidosis as well [40] (see Sect. 3.2.1).

> **Clinical Manifestation of Hypoaldosteronism**
> Dehydration, seizures (hyponatremia induced), and failure to thrive [40]

3.3.2   Cutaneous Manifestations (Folliculitis and Atopic Dermatitis)

Clinical Features
Patients with PHA1 can present with multiple cutaneous manifestations, including folliculitis and atopic dermatitis [41, 42].

Pathophysiology
Epithelial sodium chloride channels are present in multiple tissues outside the kidney, including the human skin [43]. A recent study has elucidated the role of ENaC in mediating secretions from the sebaceous glands and other eccrine glands of the skin. The inability of ENaC to mediate salt reabsorption in the sweat gland results in the accumulation of inspissated secretions in the ducts of sweat glands. This creates a suitable environment for bacterial overgrowth and inflammation (folliculitis) [41].

> **Questions You Might Be Asked on Clinical Rounds**
> *What endocrine condition can PHA type 1 be misdiagnosed as?*
>   PHA type 1 mimics an acute adrenocortical crisis in the neonatal period. Neonates will, however, not improve with glucocorticoid replacement as would be expected in patients with an adrenocortical crisis [39].
>   *How can renal (mineralocorticoid receptor gene mutation) type of PHA type 1 be differentiated from the systemic (ENaC) variant?*
>   Genetic testing and sweat gland tests [39]

3.4   Familial Glucocorticoid Deficiency

3.4.1   Hyperpigmentation

Clinical Features
Hyperpigmentation is a characteristic cutaneous sign in patients with familial glucocorticoid deficiency (FGD) [44–47], which improves with treatment [44].

Pathophysiology
ACTH stimulates *melanocortin-1 receptors* present on melanocytes of the skin. In response to this, melanocytes increase melanogenesis (hyperpigmentation) (see Sect. 3.1.2) [46].

 Pathophysiology Pearl
Pathophysiologic basis of FGD:

- FGD occurs as a result of peripheral target tissue resistance to the trophic effects of ACTH [46], due to mutations in the gene locus responsible for the translation of the *melanocortin-2 receptor (MC2R)* [44].
- ACTH is unable to bind its cognate receptor (MC2R) in the adrenal cortex, which leads to atrophy of the glucocorticoid and androgen-producing regions of the adrenal cortex. The loss of negative feedback suppression of ACTH production in the setting of hypocortisolemia promotes excess ACTH production [45].
- Mineralocorticoid action is preserved in FGD since the zone glomerulosa mediates the renin-angiotensin-aldosterone system and is not directly influenced by circulating ACTH levels [45, 46].

3.4.2   Hypoglycemia

Clinical Features
Patients with FGD can present with recurrent hypoglycemia [45, 48]. Possible hypoglycemia-related seizures have been reported [49] and can predispose patients to significant intellectual impairment [46]. Hypoglycemia should be confirmed objectively via Whipple's triad, i.e., biochemically confirmed hypoglycemia, hyperadrenergic, or neurologic symptomatology suggestive of hypoglycemia and prompt resolution of symptoms after administration of glucose (orally or parenterally) [50].

Pathophysiology
Cortisol, an essential counterregulatory hormone in glucose metabolism, is absent and predisposes patients to clinically significant hypoglycemia [44].

Questions You Might Be Asked on Clinical Rounds

What is generalized glucocorticoid resistance (GGR)?

GGR is due to a mutation in the glucocorticoid receptor gene, which results in reduced target tissue responsiveness to circulating cortisol [51]. It is indeed characterized by partial tissue resistance to the effects of cortisol [52].

What are the clinical effects of generalized glucocorticoid resistance (Chrousos syndrome)?

Due to partial pituitary insensitivity to circulating cortisol levels, there is impaired negative feedback inhibition of adrenocorticotrophic hormone (ACTH) production. Excess ACTH enhances the stimulation of the zona fasciculata and reticularis, which results in excess glucocorticoid and androgen production, respectively [53]. Excess deoxycorticosterone and corticosterone through their mineralocorticoid effects account for hypertension and hypokalemia observed in patients with this disorder. This occurs in the setting of normal circulating aldosterone. Excess androgens lead to virilization in women [52]. In boys, androgen excess may lead to early accelerated growth and muscle development followed by early epiphyseal closure and a reduced height [54] (Fig. 3.4).

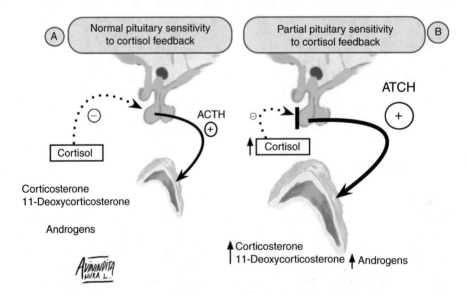

Fig. 3.4 Partial tissue insensitivity to cortisol (Chrousos syndrome). Pituitary ACTH secretion is under negative feedback control from adrenal-derived cortisol in normal physiology (**a**) [51]. Partial pituitary insensitivity to circulating cortisol levels results in increased ACTH production and eventual adrenocortical hyperplasia [52]. This accounts for the increased production of androgens, cortisol, and mineralocorticoids (11-deoxycorticosterone and corticosterone) [53, 54](**b**). (Redrawn and modified from Chrousos et al. [54])

3.5 Pheochromocytomas and Other Paraganglioma Syndromes

3.5.1 Hypertension

Clinical Features

Hypertension is the most frequent physical manifestation of pheochromocytoma, accounting for a prevalence of 80–90% in this patient population. Hypertension may be either paroxysmal or sustained, although normotension may be a presenting future in a small subset of patients [55]. Recent evidence suggests that pheochromocytomas and paraganglioma syndromes (PPGLs) account for 0.2 to 0.6% of all hypertensive cases seen in outpatient practices [56].

Pathophysiology

Direct effects of catecholamines on adrenergic and dopaminergic receptors present on cardiovascular target sites account for hypertension in patients with PPGLs [55]. See Table 3.4 for the various cardiac effects of catecholamines.

Table 3.4 Review of the location and cardiac effects of catecholamines

Adrenergic receptor (location)	Cardiac-specific effects
α1 adrenergic receptor (smooth muscle of arteries and veins)	Increases systemic blood pressure through vasoconstriction
	Positive inotropic effects [55]
α2 adrenergic receptor (presynaptic surface of sympathetic ganglia and on smooth muscles)	Arterial vasodilation [55]
β1 adrenergic receptors in cardiomyocytes	Positive inotropic effects under direct stimulation by epinephrine and norepinephrine [55]
	Positive chronotropic effects through stimulation of the cardiac pacemaker cells [55]
	Receptors present in the juxtaglomerular cells of the kidney under stimulation by catecholamines release renin leading to activation of the renin-angiotensin-aldosterone axis [55]
β2 adrenergic receptors (smooth muscles and sympathetic ganglia)	Vasodilation of muscular arteries
	Induces increased norepinephrine release from sympathetic ganglia [55]
D1 dopaminergic receptor (kidney vasculature) ⊕	Stimulation results in vasodilation of renal arteries [55]
D2 dopaminergic receptor (presynaptic) ⊕	Negative inotropic effect by inhibiting norepinephrine secretion from sympathetic nerve terminals [55]

⊕At high concentrations of dopamine, as might occur with PPGLs, dopamine stimulates α1 and β1 adrenergic receptors, which leads to vasoconstriction and an increased heart rate, respectively
Adapted from Zuber et al. [55]

☀ **Pathophysiology Pearl**

Catecholamine-Induced Hyperglycemia

1. Hyperglycemia in the setting of PPGLs occurs because of the inhibitory effect of catecholamines on insulin secretion. Binding of catecholamines, especially epinephrine to the α2 adrenergic receptor present on pancreatic beta-cells, is a widely reported mechanism [57, 58].
2. Other adrenergic effects include the induction of both hepatic gluconeogenesis and lipolysis [57].

Catecholamine Synthesis (Fig. 3.5)

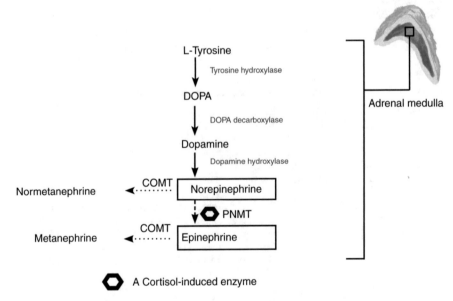

Fig. 3.5 Schematic diagram of catecholamine synthesis. The rate-limiting step in the synthesis of catecholamine occurs at the initial conversion of L-tyrosine into L-3,4-dihydroxyphenylalanine (DOPA) via the tyrosine hydroxylase enzyme. DOPA is subsequently converted to dopamine. Dopamine is hydroxylated into L-norepinephrine, which is then converted into epinephrine. The conversion of norepinephrine to epinephrine requires the cortisol-induced enzyme, phenylethanolamine-N-methyl transferase (PNMT) (dashed arrow) [55]. This is the reason why epinephrine and its metabolite (metanephrine) are only produced by PNMT-containing organs such as chromaffin cells in the adrenal gland and the organ of Zuckerkandl (located at the aortic bifurcation). Norepinephrine and epinephrine are converted into their metabolites, i.e., normetanephrine and metanephrine, respectively, by catechol-O-methyltransferase (COMT) (dotted arrow) [59]. (Based on Grouzmann et al. [59])

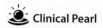 **Clinical Pearl**

Catecholamines and Fractionated Metanephrines (Understanding Terminology)

1. Continuous intratumoral conversion of *catecholamines* (epinephrine and norepinephrine) into their metabolites (metanephrine and normetanephrine, respectively) by COMT makes fractionated metanephrines either in plasma or urine a valuable screening tool. Catecholamines are, however, released intermittently; as such, screening tests involving the use of only catecholamines might miss a PPGL [60].
2. The term *fractionated metanephrines* refers to the metabolites of epinephrine and norepinephrine; these are metanephrine and normetanephrine, respectively [61].
3. Clinically significant elevation of epinephrine or metanephrine (its metabolite) almost always implies the presence of adrenal pheochromocytoma. PNMT, a cortisol-induced enzyme, although present in extra-adrenal tissues like paraganglia, is not under paracrine stimulation by cortisol in these tissues and, therefore, does not convert norepinephrine into epinephrine [62].

3.5.2 Hypotension

Clinical Features

Hypotension is usually an unexpected finding in patients with pheochromocytoma. Clinicians should, however, be aware of the possibility of a paradoxical decrease in blood pressure in patients with PPGLs [63]. Interestingly there are even reports of hypotension and hypertension rarely coexisting in rapid cycling paroxysms [64].

Pathophysiology

1. Prolonged activation of adrenergic receptors causes profound arterial and venous vasoconstriction. This process results in a reduction in cardiac output (hypotension), which is sensed by baroreceptors, leading to a compensatory increase in catecholamine release. This catecholamine surge causes sustained hypertension, which invariably activates the baroreceptor reflex arc again, leading to hypotension [65].
2. Sustained hyperstimulation of catecholamine receptors promotes their down-regulation, following which there is hypotension during periods of low catecholamine secretion [66, 67].

3.5.3   Generalized Hyperhidrosis

Clinical Features
Excessive sweating (hyperhidrosis) is a classic finding in pheochromocytoma. There is no reported prevalence in patients with pheochromocytomas, although the triad of hypertension, palpitations, and hyperhidrosis has a specificity of more than 90% in clinching the diagnosis [68].

Pathophysiology
Cholinergic input to the pilosebaceous units is responsible for their secretory output (this is independent of circulating catecholamines). Catecholamine surges during acute exacerbations of PPGLs lead to cutaneous vasoconstriction, which reduces the rate of evaporation of accumulated sweat on the skin. Indeed there is evidence that topical cholinergic blockers can prevent sweat accumulation, even in the setting of a sympathoadrenal etiology of hyperhidrosis [69].

 Pathophysiology Pearl
Hyperhidrosis, irrespective of the underlying cause, is mediated by the effects of cholinergic innervation on the sweat glands. It is essential to bear in mind that the sympathoadrenal system is not directly involved in sweat gland secretions [69].

3.5.4   Cardiogenic Shock

Clinical Features
Pheochromocytomas can cause secondary Takotsubo cardiomyopathy [70]. This classically presents with heart failure signs or even profound cardiogenic shock [71].

Pathophysiology
- Chronic stimulation of myocardial $\beta 1$ adrenergic receptors results in significant downregulation of these receptors. This, in effect, desensitizes the myocardial cells to catecholamines [67].
- Excessive levels of catecholamines increase the permeability of the myocardial sarcolemma to calcium influx. This leads to increased levels of calcium in the cytosol of the cardiac muscle and ultimately initiates a cascade of intracellular processes, which are followed by irreversible myocardial necrosis and fibrosis [67].
- Catecholamine surges in the setting of pheochromocytomas cause intense stimulation of the α and β adrenergic receptors, leading to vasoconstriction and coronary vasospasm [67].

 Clinical Pearl
PPGL is an umbrella term for both pheochromocytomas and paragangliomas. The term *pheochromocytoma* refers exclusively to tumors within the *adrenal medulla*, while the term *paraganglioma* refers to tumors *involving sympathetic and parasympathetic ganglia* [59].

Questions You Might Be Asked on Clinical Rounds

Which genetic conditions are associated with pheochromocytomas [72]?

Sporadic causes of pheochromocytomas account for most cases seen in practice. Up to a quarter of the cases have a genetic basis, which may include any of the following:

1. Multiple endocrine neoplasia (MEN) type 2A and 2B [72]
2. Von Hippel-Lindau disease (VHL) [72]
3. Neurofibromatosis type 1 (NF1) [72]

What clinical features should prompt a clinician to screen a patient for pheochromocytoma and paraganglioma syndromes (PPGLs)?

1. Adrenal incidentaloma, even in normotensive subjects [56]
2. Previous history of PPGL [56]
3. Signs and symptoms suggestive of PPGL, especially if paroxysmal [56]
4. Clinical features suggestive of the possibility of a hereditary etiology of PPGL (e.g., MEN type 2, NF1 and VHL) [56]
5. Hypertensive crises after exposure to drugs associated with PPGL-related crises (e.g., metoclopramide, beta-blockers, opioids, corticosteroids, glucagon, and neuromuscular blocking agents) [56]

3.6 Nonclassic Congenital Adrenal Hyperplasia (NCCAH)

3.6.1 Clinical Hyperandrogenism (Acne and Hirsutism)

Clinical Features

NCCAH accounts for up to 2% of cases of hyperandrogenemia involving women in their reproductive years [73]. Hirsutism, which is the growth of terminal male pattern hair, is evaluated with the modified Ferriman-Gallwey score, which happens to be a somewhat objective clinical assessment tool. There is wide variability in the prevalence of hirsutism, ranging from 1 to 33% [74].

The degree of hirsutism, however, does not correlate positively with circulating androgen levels due to differences in skin sensitivity to circulating androgens [75].

Pathophysiology
1. Most patients with NCCAH due to 21 hydroxylase deficiency typically have normal ACTH levels, in contrast to the high ACTH seen in the classic form. There is, however, excessive production of androgens in response to normal ACTH stimulation of the zona reticularis. This has been attributed to a missense mutation in the CYP21A2 gene, which results in a significant buildup of

androgen precursor steroids, due to reduced activity of the 21-hydroxylase enzyme [76]. There is an increased production of metabolites, such as DHEA-S, androstenedione, and testosterone [77]. High circulating androgens account for the acne and hirsutism seen in NCCAH [76]. *(See Sect. 1.1.4 for androgen-mediated hirsutism; see Sect. 6.2.3 for androgen-mediated acne formation.)*

2. The elevated levels of adrenal steroids impair negative feedback control of progesterone on the hypothalamic-pituitary-ovarian axis. This causes hypersecretion of LH due to rapid GnRH pulse frequency, akin to what has been proposed for the polycystic ovarian syndrome (PCOS) [78]. LH stimulates the theca cells of the ovaries to increase ovarian androgen production [76, 79].

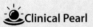**Clinical Pearl**
Other Features of Hyperandrogenemia Seen in NCCAH
    Androgenic alopecia, anovulation, and irregular menstruation [74]

3.6.2   Testicular Adrenal Rest Tumors

Clinical Features
Testicular adrenal rest tumors (TARTs) typically occur in males with classical congenital adrenal hyperplasia, although it has been reported in NCCAH as well [80]. TARTs in boys with congenital adrenal hyperplasia (CAH) are known to regress in size with optimal supplementation of hormonal insufficiencies. They are diagnosed based on clinical and radiographic findings, with biopsies being unnecessary in most cases [81].

Pathophysiology
Adrenal and gonadal cells are located adjacent to each other in the developing embryo. Inadvertent translocation of embryonic adrenal cells to the gonads occurs during gonadal descent. The lack of atrophy of these ectopic adrenal tissues in the setting of NCCAH or CAH is the cause of TARTs [81]. ACTH binds to ACTH receptors present on adrenal tissue in the testes, and this trophic stimulation of the ectopic adrenal tissue by ACTH results in their growth [82].

3.6.3   Signs of Insulin Resistance (Skin Tags and Acanthosis Nigricans)

Clinical Features
Insulin resistance has a significant association with NCCAH [83, 84], although some authors believe this association could be secondary to glucocorticoid use in this patient population [76, 85]. Hyperinsulinemia-mediated skin manifestations have been described elsewhere. (See Sect. 4.1.3 for acrochordons and Sect. 4.1.1 for acanthosis nigricans.)

Pathophysiology

The mechanisms underlying hyperinsulinemia in NCCAH are incompletely under-stood [84, 86].

Normalization of serum androgen does not ameliorate insulin resistance, making hyperandrogenemia an unlikely cause of insulin resistance in patients with NCCAH [87].

 Clinical Pearl

Choice of Steroid Replacement Therapy in Pregnant Patients with NCCAH

Exposure of the fetal brain to exogenous steroids can cause intellectual impairment. Dexamethasone crosses the placenta since it is not metabolized by placental 11 beta-hydroxysteroid dehydrogenase type 2 (11BSD2). Prednisone and hydrocortisone, on the other hand, are metabolized by 11BHSD2 and, as such, preferred in pregnancy [76].

 Questions You Might Be Asked on Clinical Rounds

What are the genetic differences between NCCAH and the classic congenital adrenal hyperplasia (Table 3.5)?

What are the various clinicopathologic phenotypes of congenital adrenal hyperplasia (CAH)?

The primary defect in CAH is an adrenal steroidogenic enzyme defect, which results in low levels of serum cortisol. The loss of negative feedback control activates the hypothalamic-pituitary-adrenal axis, which results in increased adrenocorticotropic hormone (ACTH) production. ACTH stimulates the buildup and subsequent shunting of precursor steroids into either androgen or mineralocorticoid production [75].

A brief review of the adrenal steroidogenesis pathway is critical in appreciating the various clinicopathologic phenotypes of CAH (Fig. 3.6).

Table 3.5   Comparison of CAH and NCCAH

CAH	NCCAH
Large gene deletion involving the CYP21A2 gene	Usually, a point mutation (70% of patients) in the CYP21A2 gene [85]
Loss of 21-hydroxylase enzyme activity by 95–100%	Loss of 21-hydroxylase enzyme activity by 20–50% [85]

Adapted from Trapp et al. [85]

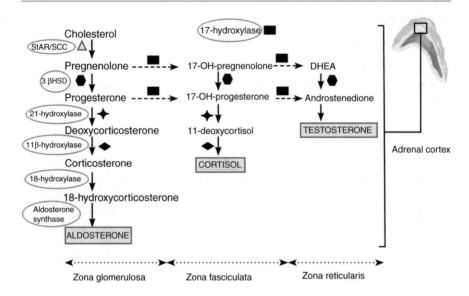

Fig. 3.6 Steroidogenic pathway depicting the various enzyme defects in congenital adrenal hyperplasia. The steroidogenic acute regulatory protein (StAR), at the level of the adrenal gland, mobilizes cholesterol from the outer to the inner mitochondrial membrane. The cytochrome P450 side-cleavage enzyme (P450scc) in the inner mitochondrial membrane converts cholesterol to pregnenolone; this is the rate-limiting step of adrenal steroidogenesis. The downstream effects of StAR are under trophic stimulation by both ACTH and luteinizing hormone (LH) [88]. Pregnenolone is then converted to the progesterone by 3beta-hydroxysteroid dehydrogenase type 2 (HSD3B2), in the zona glomerulosa. Progesterone is then converted through a series of enzymatic steps involving 21 hydroxylase (CYP21A2) and aldosterone synthase into aldosterone. In the zona fasciculata, pregnenolone is hydroxylated into 17-hydroxypregnenolone by CYP17A1 (17-alpha-hydroxylase enzyme/17,20 lyase). HSD3B2, CYP21A2, and CYP11B1 (11 beta-hydroxylase) are then involved in downstream reactions leading to the production of cortisol. In the zona reticularis, CYP17A1 and HSD3B2 are involved in the eventual formation of androgen precursors such as dehydroepiandrosterone (DHEA) and androstenedione [89]. (Redrawn and modified from Al Alawi et al. [89])

Phenotypes of Congenital Adrenal Hyperplasia

1. *Congenital lipoid hyperplasia (CLH).* CLH is due to an autosomal recessive mutation in the gene encoding StAR. Clinical features include severe adrenal insufficiency (both mineralocorticoid and glucocorticoid deficiency) and external female genitalia in male infants. It is a fatal form of CAH [90].
2. *3Beta-hydroxysteroid dehydrogenase type 2 deficiency.* The clinical spectrum of 3BHSD varies from a presentation akin to CLH (both mineralocorticoid and glucocorticoid deficiency) to an even less severe subtype characterized by the absence of salt-wasting [91].
3. *17 hydroxylase deficiency.* A genetic mutation in CYP17A1 impairs steroidogenesis in both the adrenal glands and gonads [92]. Genetic females have normal-appearing female external genitalia at birth but subsequently present with delayed puberty. Male infants, on the other hand, are unable to synthesize

testosterone, critical in developing male external genitalia. This results in the formation of female appearing external genitalia [93, 94]. Also, males do not have internal Mullerian structures (uterus and fallopian tubes) since their anatomic testes continue to produce anti-Mullerian hormone (see Sect. 6.6.1). Despite patients being mildly glucocorticoid deficient, they seldom develop overt adrenal crises. This is because of the accumulation of precursors such as corticosterone and 11-deoxycorticosterone (DOC) not only activates the mineralocorticoid receptor to maintain blood pressure but also contributes to hypertension in affected patients [95].

4. *11 beta-hydroxylase deficiency.* A genetic mutation in CYP11B1 results in a defective 11beta hydroxylase, a critical enzyme in cortisol synthesis [96, 97]. There is, therefore, an accumulation of proximal precursors such as DOC and 11-deoxycortisol. DOC has intrinsic mineralocorticoid activity and accounts for hypertension and hypokalemia observed in these patients [98]. There is an additional shunting of more proximal steroids into androgen production (DHEA, DHEA-S, and androstenedione). Genetic males have enlarged penile shafts at birth due to hyperandrogenemia. Genetic females have ambiguous genitalia due to exposure to elevated serum androgens during intrauterine life [98, 99].

5. *21 hydroxylase deficiency.* A genetic mutation in CYP21A2 results in a defective 21 hydroxylase enzyme. 21-Hydroxylation of progesterone (mineralocorticoid synthesis pathway) and 17-hydroxyprogesterone (glucocorticoid synthesis pathway) is therefore impaired. There is a subsequent diversion of proximal steroidogenic precursors into androgen production. Newborns with more deleterious mutations in the CYP21A2 gene are hemodynamically unstable due to impaired glucocorticoid and mineralocorticoid synthesis. Genetic females present with ambiguous genitalia [100].

References

1. Burton C, Cottrell E, Edwards J. Addison's disease: identification and management in primary care. Br J Gen Pract. 2015;65:488–90.
2. Papierska L, Rabijewski M. Delay in diagnosis of adrenal insufficiency is a frequent cause of adrenal crisis. Int J Endocrinol. 2013;2013:482370.
3. Hellesen A, Bratland E, Husebye ES. Autoimmune Addison's disease – an update on pathogenesis. Ann Endocrinol. 2018;79:157–63.
4. Letizia C, Cerci S, Centanni M, De Toma G, Subioli S, Scuro L, Scavo D. Circulating levels of adrenomedullin in patients with Addison's disease before and after corticosteroid treatment. Clin Endocrinol. 1998;48:145–8.
5. Ullian ME. The role of corticosteroids in the regulation of vascular tone. Cardiovasc Res. 1999;41:55–64.
6. Barajas L. Anatomy of the juxtaglomerular apparatus. Am J Phys. 1979;237:F333–43.
7. Martini AG, Danser AHJ. Juxtaglomerular cell phenotypic plasticity. High Blood Press Cardiovasc Prev. 2017;24:231–42.
8. Peti-Peterdi J, Harris RC. Macula Densa sensing and signaling mechanisms of renin release. J Am Soc Nephrol JASN. 2010;21:1093–6.

9. Durante A, Peretto G, Laricchia A, Ancona F, Spartera M, Mangieri A, Cianflone D. Role of the renin-angiotensin-aldosterone system in the pathogenesis of atherosclerosis. Curr Pharm Des. 2012;18:981–1004.
10. Oelkers W, Diederich S, Bähr V. Diagnosis and therapy surveillance in Addison's disease: rapid adrenocorticotropin (ACTH) test and measurement of plasma ACTH, renin activity, and aldosterone. J Clin Endocrinol Metab. 1992;75:259–64.
11. Kumar R, Kumari S, Ranabijuli PK. Generalized pigmentation due to Addison disease. Dermatol Online J. 2008;14:13.
12. Yamamoto H, Yamane T, Iguchi K, Tanaka K, Iddamalgoda A, Unno K, Hoshino M, Takeda A. Melanin production through novel processing of proopiomelanocortin in the extracellular compartment of the auricular skin of C57BL/6 mice after UV-irradiation. Sci Rep. 2015;5:14579.
13. Pramanik S, Bhattacharjee R, Mukhopadhyay P, Ghosh S. Lesson of the month 2: Houssay phenomenon – hypopituitarism leading to remission of diabetes. Clin Med. 2016;16:294–6.
14. Cesmebasi A, Plessis MD, Iannatuono M, Shah S, Tubbs RS, Loukas M. A review of the anatomy and clinical significance of adrenal veins. Clin Anat. 2014;27:1253–63.
15. Kahn SL, Angle JF. Adrenal Vein Sampling. Tech Vasc Interv Radiol. 2010;13:110–25.
16. Park J, Didi M, Blair J. The diagnosis and treatment of adrenal insufficiency during childhood and adolescence. Arch Dis Child. 2016;101:860–5.
17. Mandadi S, Sattar S, Towfiq B, Bachuwa G. A case of nausea and vomiting to remember. BMJ Case Rep. 2015; https://doi.org/10.1136/bcr-2014-207251.
18. Auron M, Raissouni N. Adrenal insufficiency. Pediatr Rev. 2015;36:92.
19. Brian BJ, Turcu AF, Auchus RJ. Primary Aldosteronism. Circulation. 2018;138:823–35.
20. Ong GSY, Young MJ. Mineralocorticoid regulation of cell function: the role of rapid signalling and gene transcription pathways. J Mol Endocrinol. 2017;58:R33–57.
21. Valinsky WC, Touyz RM. Shrier a (2018) aldosterone, SGK1, and ion channels in the kidney. Clin Sci Lond Engl. 1979;132:173–83.
22. Wu C, Xin J, Xin M, Zou H, Jing L, Zhu C, Lei W. Hypokalemic myopathy in primary aldosteronism: a case report. Exp Ther Med. 2016;12:4064–6.
23. Kotsaftis P, Savopoulos C, Agapakis D, Ntaios G, Tzioufa V, Papadopoulos V, Fahantidis E, Hatzitolios A. Hypokalemia induced myopathy as first manifestation of primary hyperaldosteronism - an elderly patient with unilateral adrenal hyperplasia: a case report. Cases J. 2009;2:6813.
24. Olt S, Yaylaci S, Tatli L, Gunduz Y, Garip T, Tamer A. Hypokalemia- induced myopathy and massive creatine kinase elevation as first manifestation of Conn's syndrome. Niger Med J J Niger Med Assoc. 2013;54:283–4.
25. Seccia TM, Caroccia B, Adler G, Maiolino G, Cesari M. Rossi GP (2017) arterial hypertension, atrial fibrillation and hyperaldosteronism: the triple trouble. Hypertens Dallas Tex. 1979;69:545–50.
26. Paolo RG, Giuseppe M, Alberto F, et al. Adrenalectomy lowers incident atrial fibrillation in primary Aldosteronism patients at long term. Hypertension. 2018;71:585–91.
27. Julian H, Charle V, Ashley C. Irregular, narrow-complex tachycardia. Cardiovasc J Afr. 2018;29:195–8.
28. Kim K, Lee JH, Kim SC, Cha DR, Kang YS. A case of primary aldosteronism combined with acquired nephrogenic diabetes insipidus. Kidney Res Clin Pract. 2014;33:229–33.
29. Marples D, Frøkiaer J, Dørup J, Knepper MA, Nielsen S. Hypokalemia-induced downregulation of aquaporin-2 water channel expression in rat kidney medulla and cortex. J Clin Invest. 1996;97:1960–8.
30. Schrier RW. Aldosterone "escape" vs "breakthrough". Nat Rev Nephrol. 2010;6:61.
31. Funder JW, Carey RM, Mantero F, Murad MH, Reincke M, Shibata H, Stowasser M, Young WF. The Management of Primary Aldosteronism: case detection, diagnosis, and treatment: an Endocrine Society clinical practice guideline. J Clin Endocrinol Metab. 2016;101:1889–916.
32. Sabbadin C, Armanini D. Syndromes that mimic an excess of mineralocorticoids. High Blood Press Cardiovasc Prev. 2016;23:231–5.

33. Tetti M, Monticone S, Burrello J, Matarazzo P, Veglio F, Pasini B, Jeunemaitre X, Mulatero P. Liddle syndrome: review of the literature and description of a new case. Int J Mol Sci. 2018; https://doi.org/10.3390/ijms19030812.

34. O'Shaughnessy KM. Gordon syndrome: a continuing story. Pediatr Nephrol Berl Ger. 2015;30:1903–8.

35. Young William F. Chapter 16 - Endocrine Hypertension. In: Melmed S, Polonsky KS, Larsen PR, Kronenberg HM, editors. Williams Textb. Endocrinol. 13th ed. Philadelphia: Content Repository Only! 2016. p. 556–88.

36. Armanini D, Calò L, Semplicini A. Pseudohyperaldosteronism: pathogenetic mechanisms. Crit Rev Clin Lab Sci. 2003;40:295–335.

37. Al-Harbi T, Al-Shaikh A. Apparent mineralocorticoid excess syndrome: report of one family with three affected children. J Pediatr Endocrinol Metab JPEM. 2012;25:1083–8.

38. Attia NA, Marzouk YI. Pseudohypoaldosteronism in a neonate presenting as life-threatening hyperkalemia. Case Rep Endocrinol. 2016; https://doi.org/10.1155/2016/6384697.

39. Amin N, Alvi NS, Barth JH, et al. Pseudohypoaldosteronism type 1: clinical features and management in infancy. Endocrinol Diabetes Metab Case Rep. 2013;2013:130010.

40. Bizzarri C, Olivini N, Pedicelli S, Marini R, Giannone G, Cambiaso P, Cappa M. Congenital primary adrenal insufficiency and selective aldosterone defects presenting as salt-wasting in infancy: a single center 10-year experience. Ital J Pediatr. 2016;42:73.

41. Hanukoglu I, Boggula VR, Vaknine H, Sharma S, Kleyman T, Hanukoglu A. Expression of epithelial sodium channel (ENaC) and CFTR in the human epidermis and epidermal appendages. Histochem Cell Biol. 2017;147:733–48.

42. Hanukoglu A, Hanukoglu I. In systemic pseudohypoaldosteronism type 1 skin manifestations are not rare and the disease is not transient. Clin Endocrinol. 2018;89:240–1.

43. Yamamura H, Ugawa S, Ueda T, Shimada S. Expression analysis of the epithelial Na+ channel delta subunit in human melanoma G-361 cells. Biochem Biophys Res Commun. 2008;366:489–92.

44. Metwalley KA, Farghaly HS. Familial glucocorticoid deficiency presenting with generalized hyperpigmentation in an Egyptian child: a case report. J Med Case Rep. 2012;6:110.

45. Jacoby E, Barzilai A, Laufer J, Pade S, Anikster Y, Pinhas-Hamiel O, Greenberger S. Neonatal hyperpigmentation: diagnosis of familial glucocorticoid deficiency with a novel mutation in the melanocortin-2 receptor gene. Pediatr Dermatol. 2014;31:e13–7.

46. Jneibi FA, Hen T, Rajah J, Nair R. Early diagnosis in familial glucocorticoid deficiency. Dermatoendocrinol. 2017;9:e1310787.

47. Akın L, Kurtoğlu S, Kendirici M, Akın MA. Familial glucocorticoid deficiency type 2: a case report. J Clin Res Pediatr Endocrinol. 2010;2:122–5.

48. Chung T-TLL, Chan LF, Metherell LA, Clark AJL. Phenotypic characteristics of familial glucocorticoid deficiency (FGD) type 1 and 2. Clin Endocrinol. 2010;72:589–94.

49. Modan-Moses D, Ben-Zeev B, Hoffmann C, Falik-Zaccai TC, Bental YA, Pinhas-Hamiel O, Anikster Y. Unusual presentation of familial glucocorticoid deficiency with a novel MRAP mutation. J Clin Endocrinol Metab. 2006;91:3713–7.

50. Miron I, Diaconescu S, Aprodu G, Ioniuc I, Diaconescu MR, Miron L. Diagnostic difficulties in a pediatric Insulinoma: a case report. Medicine (Baltimore). 2016;95:e3045.

51. Charmandari E, Kino T, Ichijo T, Chrousos GP. Generalized glucocorticoid resistance: clinical aspects, molecular mechanisms, and implications of a rare genetic disorder. J Clin Endocrinol Metab. 2008;93:1563–72.

52. Charmandari E, Kino T, Chrousos GP. Primary generalized familial and sporadic glucocorticoid resistance (Chrousos syndrome) and hypersensitivity. Endocr Dev. 2013;24:67–85.

53. Nicolaides NC, Charmandari E. Chrousos syndrome: from molecular pathogenesis to therapeutic management. Eur J Clin Investig. 2015;45:504–14.

54. Chrousos GP, Detera-Wadleigh SD, Karl M. Syndromes of glucocorticoid resistance. Ann Intern Med. 1993;119:1113–24.

55. Zuber SM, Kantorovich V, Pacak K. Hypertension in Pheochromocytoma: characteristics and treatment. Endocrinol Metab Clin N Am. 2011;40:295–311.

56. Lenders JWM, Duh Q-Y, Eisenhofer G, Gimenez-Roqueplo A-P, Grebe SKG, Murad MH, Naruse M, Pacak K, Young WF. Pheochromocytoma and Paraganglioma: an Endocrine Society clinical practice guideline. J Clin Endocrinol Metab. 2014;99:1915–42.
57. Lee I-S, Lee T-W, Chang C-J, Chien Y-M, Lee T-I. Pheochromocytoma presenting as hyperglycemic hyperosmolar syndrome and unusual fever. Intern Emerg Med. 2015;10:753–5.
58. Debuyser A, Drews G, Henquin JC. Adrenaline inhibition of insulin release: role of the repolarization of the B cell membrane. Pflüg Arch. 1991;419:131–7.
59. Grouzmann E, Tschopp O, Triponez F, et al. Catecholamine metabolism in Paraganglioma and Pheochromocytoma: similar tumors in different sites? PLoS One. 2015;10:e0125426.
60. Grouzmann E, Drouard-Troalen L, Baudin E, Plouin P-F, Muller B, Grand D, Buclin T. Diagnostic accuracy of free and total metanephrines in plasma and fractionated metanephrines in urine of patients with pheochromocytoma. Eur J Endocrinol. 2010;162:951–60.
61. Kim HJ, Lee JI, Cho YY, et al. Diagnostic accuracy of plasma free metanephrines in a seated position compared with 24-hour urinary metanephrines in the investigation of pheochromocytoma. Endocr J. 2015;62:243–50.
62. Kantorovich V, Pacak K. Pheochromocytoma and paraganglioma. Prog Brain Res. 2010;182:343–73.
63. Mabulac MP, Abad LR. Pheochromocytoma presenting as hypotension in a 12 year old female. Int J Pediatr Endocrinol. 2013;2013:P117.
64. Ionescu CN, Sakharova OV, Harwood MD, Caracciolo EA, Schoenfeld MH, Donohue TJ. Cyclic rapid fluctuation of hypertension and hypotension in Pheochromocytoma. J Clin Hypertens. 2008;10:936–40.
65. Kobal SL, Paran E, Jamali A, Mizrahi S, Siegel RJ, Leor J. Pheochromocytoma: cyclic attacks of hypertension alternating with hypotension. Nat Rev Cardiol. 2008;5:53–7.
66. Shin E, Ko KS, Rhee BD, Han J, Kim N. Different effects of prolonged β-adrenergic stimulation on heart and cerebral artery. Integr Med Res. 2014;3:204–10.
67. Kassim TA, Clarke DD, Mai VQ, Clyde PW, MohamedShakir KM. Catecholamine-induced cardiomyopathy. Endocr Pract Jacksonv. 2008;14:1137–49.
68. Falhammar H, Kjellman M, Calissendorff J. Initial clinical presentation and spectrum of pheochromocytoma: a study of 94 cases from a single center. Endocr Connect. 2017;7:186–92.
69. Robertshaw D. Hyperhidrosis and the sympatho-adrenal system. Med Hypotheses. 1979;5:317–22.
70. Chiang Y-L, Chen P-C, Lee C-C, Chua S-K. Adrenal pheochromocytoma presenting with Takotsubo-pattern cardiomyopathy and acute heart failure: a case report and literature review. Medicine (Baltimore). 2016;95:e4846.
71. Loscalzo J, Roy N, Shah RV, Tsai JN, Cahalane AM, Steiner J, Stone JR. Case 8-2018: a 55-year-old woman with shock and labile blood pressure. N Engl J Med. 2018;378:1043–53.
72. Alface MM, Moniz P, Jesus S, Fonseca C. Pheochromocytoma: clinical review based on a rare case in adolescence. BMJ Case Rep. 2015; https://doi.org/10.1136/bcr-2015-211184.
73. Ambroziak U, Kępczyńska-Nyk A, Kuryłowicz A, Małunowicz EM, Wójcicka A, Miśkiewicz P, Macech M. The diagnosis of nonclassic congenital adrenal hyperplasia due to 21-hydroxylase deficiency, based on serum basal or post-ACTH stimulation 17-hydroxyprogesterone, can lead to false-positive diagnosis. Clin Endocrinol. 2016;84:23–9.
74. Witchel SF, Azziz R. Nonclassic congenital adrenal hyperplasia. Int J Pediatr Endocrinol. 2010; https://doi.org/10.1155/2010/625105.
75. Witchel SF. Congenital adrenal hyperplasia. J Pediatr Adolesc Gynecol. 2017;30:520–34.
76. Carmina E, Dewailly D, Escobar-Morreale HF, Kelestimur F, Moran C, Oberfield S, Witchel SF, Azziz R. Non-classic congenital adrenal hyperplasia due to 21-hydroxylase deficiency revisited: an update with a special focus on adolescent and adult women. Hum Reprod Update. 2017;23:580–99.
77. Speiser PW, Arlt W, Auchus RJ, et al. Congenital adrenal hyperplasia due to steroid 21-hydroxylase deficiency: an Endocrine Society clinical practice guideline. J Clin Endocrinol Metab. 2018;103:4043–88.
78. Witchel SF. Non-classic congenital adrenal hyperplasia. Steroids. 2013;78:747–50.
79. Blank SK, McCartney CR, Helm KD, Marshall JC. Neuroendocrine effects of androgens in adult polycystic ovary syndrome and female puberty. Semin Reprod Med. 2007;25:352–9.

80. Kurtoğlu S, Hatipoğlu N. Non-classical congenital adrenal hyperplasia in childhood. J Clin Res Pediatr Endocrinol. 2017;9:1–7.

81. Kocova M, Janevska V, Anastasovska V. Testicular adrenal rest tumors in boys with 21-hydroxylase deficiency, timely diagnosis and follow-up. Endocr Connect. 2018;7:544–52.

82. Kim MS, Goodarzian F, Keenan MF, Geffner ME, Koppin CM, De Filippo RE, Kokorowski PJ. Testicular adrenal rest tumors in boys and Young adults with congenital adrenal hyperplasia. J Urol. 2017;197:931–6.

83. Powell D, Inoue T, Bahtiyar G, Fenteany G, Sacerdote A. Treatment of nonclassic 11-hydroxylase deficiency with Ashwagandha root. Case Rep Endocrinol. 2017; https://doi.org/10.1155/2017/1869560.

84. Saygili F, Oge A, Yilmaz C. Hyperinsulinemia and insulin insensitivity in women with non-classical congenital adrenal hyperplasia due to 21-hydroxylase deficiency: the relationship between serum leptin levels and chronic hyperinsulinemia. Horm Res. 2005;63:270–4.

85. Trapp CM, Oberfield SE. Recommendations for treatment of nonclassic congenital adrenal hyperplasia (NCCAH): an update. Steroids. 2012;77:342–6.

86. Pall M, Azziz R, Beires J, Pignatelli D. The phenotype of hirsute women: a comparison of polycystic ovary syndrome and 21-hydroxylase-deficient nonclassic adrenal hyperplasia. Fertil Steril. 2010;94:684–9.

87. Singer F, Bhargava G, Poretsky L. Persistent insulin resistance after normalization of androgen levels in a woman with congenital adrenal hyperplasia. A case report J Reprod Med. 1989;34:921–2.

88. King SR, Stocco DM. Steroidogenic acute regulatory protein expression in the central nervous system. Front Endocrinol. 2011; https://doi.org/10.3389/fendo.2011.00072.

89. Al Alawi AM, Nordenström A, Falhammar H. Clinical perspectives in congenital adrenal hyperplasia due to 3β-hydroxysteroid dehydrogenase type 2 deficiency. Endocrine. 2019;63:407–21.

90. Kim CJ. Congenital lipoid adrenal hyperplasia. Ann Pediatr Endocrinol Metab. 2014;19:179–83.

91. Sahakitrungruang T. Clinical and molecular review of atypical congenital adrenal hyperplasia. Ann Pediatr Endocrinol Metab. 2015;20:1–7.

92. Fontenele R, Costa-Santos M, Kater CE. 17α-hydroxylase deficiency is an underdiagnosed disease: high frequency of misdiagnosis in a large cohort of Brazilian patients. Endocr Pract Off J Am Coll Endocrinol Am Assoc Clin Endocrinol. 2018;24:170–8.

93. Kim SM, Rhee JH. A case of 17 alpha-hydroxylase deficiency. Clin Exp Reprod Med. 2015;42:72–6.

94. Kardelen AD, Toksoy G, Baş F, et al. A rare cause of congenital adrenal hyperplasia: clinical and genetic findings and follow-up characteristics of six patients with 17-hydroxylase deficiency including two novel mutations. J Clin Res Pediatr Endocrinol. 2018;10:206–15.

95. Auchus RJ. Steroid 17-hydroxylase and 17,20-Lyase deficiencies, genetic and pharmacologic. J Steroid Biochem Mol Biol. 2017;165:71–8.

96. White PC. Congenital adrenal hyperplasia owing to 11β-hydroxylase deficiency. Adv Exp Med Biol. 2011;707:7–8.

97. Ben Charfeddine I, Riepe FG, Kahloul N, et al. Two novel CYP11B1 mutations in congenital adrenal hyperplasia due to steroid 11β hydroxylase deficiency in a Tunisian family. Gen Comp Endocrinol. 2012;175:514–8.

98. Bulsari K, Falhammar H. Clinical perspectives in congenital adrenal hyperplasia due to 11β-hydroxylase deficiency. Endocrine. 2017;55:19–36.

99. Khattab A, Haider S, Kumar A, et al. Clinical, genetic, and structural basis of congenital adrenal hyperplasia due to 11β-hydroxylase deficiency. Proc Natl Acad Sci U S A. 2017;114:E1933–40.

100. White PC, Speiser PW. Congenital adrenal hyperplasia due to 21-hydroxylase deficiency. Endocr Rev. 2000;21:245–91.

Pancreatic Gland Signs

4

Learning Objectives
At the end of this chapter, you will be able to:

1. Discover the pathophysiologic basis for some dermatologic manifestations of hyperinsulinemia
2. Discuss the pathophysiologic basis for diabetic retinopathy and nephropathy
3. Discuss the mechanisms underlying insulin resistance in T2DM patients
4. Categorize various insulin-resistant states and determine their clinical relevance
5. Discuss the mechanisms underlying the clinical manifestations of neuro-endocrine tumors, including VIPomas, gastrinomas, insulinomas, PPomas, and glucagonomas.

4.1 Diabetes Mellitus

4.1.1 Acanthosis Nigricans

Clinical Features
Acanthosis nigricans (AN) is a hyperpigmented lesion with a predilection for flexural areas such as the neck, axilla, and intertriginous regions of the body. Patients with type 2 diabetes mellitus, an obese phenotype, or the metabolic syndrome are predisposed to developing this classic skin lesion [1].

Pathophysiology
1. Insulin activates IGF-1 receptors present on fibroblasts and keratinocytes. This is reported to be an essential mechanistic pathway involved in the development of AN. Histologically, there is evidence of hypermelanosis and hyperkeratosis.

© Springer Nature Switzerland AG 2020
A. Manni, A. Quarde, *Endocrine Pathophysiology*,
https://doi.org/10.1007/978-3-030-49872-6_4

The histological findings affirm the role of some inciting mediators involved in the proliferation of keratinocytes and fibroblasts [1].

2. Additionally, hyperinsulinemia causes a decrease in IGF-binding proteins, which results in a higher level of unbound (active) IGF-1 [1].

3. Interestingly, androgens and growth factor receptors are present on keratinocytes and fibroblasts as well. It appears these mediators may explain the presence of AN in other endocrinopathies such as polycystic ovary syndrome (PCOS), congenital adrenal hyperplasia (CAH), and acromegaly [1].

Other Endocrinopathies Associated with Acanthosis Nigricans
Cushing's syndrome; Addison's disease (see Sect. 3.1.2); PCOS; CAH; hyperandrogenism, insulin resistance, and acanthosis nigricans (HAIR-AN) syndrome; and acromegaly (see Sect. 1.2.1) [1]

4.1.2   Diabetic Dermopathy

Clinical Features
Diabetic dermopathy (DD) is reported as a cardinal skin manifestation of both type 1 and type 2 diabetes mellitus. It presents as hyperpigmented and circumscribed macules noted over the pretibial skin. These characteristic lesions have a predilection for areas prone to trauma and are present in up to 55% of patients with diabetes mellitus (DM) [2].

Pathophysiology
Neuropathy and microangiopathy induced by uncontrolled diabetes mellitus [2]

4.1.3   Acrochordons (Skin Tags)

Clinical Features
Skin tags have a reported prevalence of 25% in patients with type 2 diabetes mellitus. The lesions are pedunculated cutaneous fibromas distributed over flexural areas in the neck and axilla, in a pattern akin to the distribution of AN [3].

Pathophysiology
Endogenous hyperinsulinemia promotes the activation of fibroblast-bound IGF-1 receptors present in the epidermis. This is followed by the proliferation of skin fibroblasts and subsequent development of skin tags [2].

4.1.4   Necrobiosis Lipoidica Diabeticorum

Clinical Features
Necrobiosis lipoidica diabeticorum (NLD) is a rare clinical finding in patients with either type 1 or type 2 diabetes mellitus. The lesions typically start as a red-brown

papule that progressively increases in diameter and eventually changes into the classic waxy, yellowish lesion. There is an occasional central ulceration, which manifests as an atrophic center [4].

Pathophysiology
There is initial tissue hypoperfusion in the skin due to microangiopathy involving skin capillaries. Microangiopathy occurs as a result of the accumulation of advanced glycation end products in the vasculature, which consequently promotes local oxidative stress. Inflammatory mediators which have accumulated in response to tissue hypoperfusion lead to a progressive breakdown in collagen [4].

4.1.5 Lipodystrophy Due to Insulin Injections

Clinical Features
Localized lipodystrophy due to insulin injections is an umbrella term which consists of the lipoatrophy (LA) and lipohypertrophy (LH) subtypes [5].

LA tends to appear as an area of subcutaneous tissue loss, which creates a dimple in the skin. LH, however, has a firm, rubbery consistency that is palpable in the subcutaneous tissue plane. Occasionally, LH lesions may be soft, making them difficult to discern on routine physical examination [5]. Ultrasound is more sensitive than the clinical exam for the detection of lipodystrophy. Lipodystrophic areas can lead to malabsorption of insulin (either delayed or more rapid) from the subcutaneous tissue. This reportedly causes wide variability in glycemic control and can drastically impact patient care if it remains undiagnosed [6].

In a meta-analysis of over 12,000 patients with diabetes mellitus, the pooled prevalence estimate of lipodystrophy was astonishingly high at 38% (95% confidence interval 29–46%). LH is best appreciated clinically by palpating the affected area with the pulp of the fingertips [7].

Pathophysiology
1. Lipoatrophy occurs as a result of an immune-mediated reaction to insulin; it is less prevalent now, due to the use of modern human insulin or humanlike insulin analogs [5].
2. Lipohypertrophy is due to the growth-promoting effects of insulin on fibroblasts in the subcutaneous tissue. Insulin binds to IGF-1 receptors on fibroblasts. Such binding leads to the activation and subsequent proliferation of fibroblasts [5].

There are a host of other cutaneous manifestations of DM, well beyond the scope of this text. Some selected skin manifestations and their pathophysiologic basis are reviewed in Table 4.1.

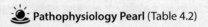
Pathophysiology Pearl (Table 4.2)

Table 4.1 Other skin manifestations of diabetes mellitus

Lesion	Clinical findings	Pathophysiology
Eruptive xanthoma	Yellowish papules located over the trunk and extensor surfaces such as the elbows and knees	Reduced lipoprotein lipase activity due to insulin resistance or insulinopenia causes impaired storage of triglycerides in adipose tissue (see Sect. 1.4.1). Following which excess circulating triglycerides accumulate in the skin [3]
Bullosis diabeticorum	Usually located on the lower extremities. Bullae tend to contain a clear fluid which can be aspirated when it causes discomfort	Unknown [3]
Scleroderma diabeticorum	Thick, indurated plaques tend to be distributed over the neck and upper back	Reduced breakdown of collagen fibers due to nonenzymatic glycosylation of dermal collagen [3]
Granuloma annulare	Firm, erythematous papules with a ringlike configuration	Microangiopathy, lymphocytic infiltration, and eventual connective tissue degeneration [8]

Adapted from Duff [3] and Thornsberry [8]

Table 4.2 Pathophysiologic basis of some forms of diabetes mellitus

Type of diabetes	Pathophysiology
Type 1 diabetes mellitus (T1DM)	Immune-mediated destruction of pancreatic beta-cells [9]
Type 2 diabetes mellitus (T2DM)	Reduction in incretin effect, suppression of insulin secretion, increased lipolysis, increased renal conservation of glucose, increased gluconeogenesis, reduced peripheral utilization of glucose (muscle and adipose tissue), increased glucagon secretion and central neurotransmitter dysfunction (hyperphagia) [10][a]
Gestational diabetes mellitus (GDM)	The physiology of pregnancy (increased food intake, placental counterregulatory hormones, and a gain of adipose tissue) contributes to pancreatic beta-cell dysfunction and peripheral insulin resistance [11]
Cystic fibrosis-related diabetes (CFRD)	Cystic fibrosis transmembrane conductance regulator (CFTR) modulates both pancreatic beta- and alpha-cell function, by altering multiple electrolyte channels involved in hormone secretion [12]
Posttransplant diabetes mellitus (PTDM)	Immunosuppressive therapy (glucocorticoid-induced hyperglycemia, calcineurin modulators, mTOR modulators) [13]
Pancreatogenic diabetes (type 3c DM) (pancreoprivic diabetes) [14]	Anatomic loss of pancreatic beta-cell function (pancreatectomy, chronic pancreatitis, infiltrative tumors) [15]
Maturity-onset diabetes of the young (MODY)	Single gene mutation which impairs insulin secretion [16]. There are at least 13 identified genes, thus far [17]
Latent autoimmune diabetes in adulthood (LADA)	Immune-mediated destruction of pancreatic beta-cells, akin to T1DM, albeit at a much slower pace [18]

[a]This is classically referred to as the "the ominous octet," a term coined by Dr. Ralph DeFronzo, *mTOR* mammalian target of rapamycin
Adapted from Refs. [9–18]

> :sunny: **Clinical Pearl**
>
> *Mucormycosis in the Setting of Diabetic Ketoacidosis (DKA)*
>   *Mucormycosis* is caused by at least six different families of fungi, including *Rhizopus* species. Patients in DKA are at risk of developing this life-threatening infection [19]. It classically appears as a dark eschar involving the oral palate and may, in some circumstances, progress into the nose and brain (rhinocerebral mucormycosis). Extraoral sites of infection include the skin, lung, and gastrointestinal tract [20].

Pathophysiology
- Hyperglycemia and ketoacidosis impair the activity of neutrophils critical in fighting this fungal infection.
- Rhizopus species are "iron-loving" or ferrophilic fungi. An acidotic state, as occurs in DKA, increases the amount of free iron available for the fungus to grow by reducing the binding of iron to transferrin (an iron-binding protein) [19].

4.1.6 Diabetic Retinopathy on Direct Ophthalmoscopy

Clinical Features
The direct ophthalmoscope, an essential component of the physical exam, is increasingly not being utilized by present-day physicians. Recent evidence points to an increasing trend of low competency in the use of direct the ophthalmoscope [21]. Nonetheless, direct ophthalmoscopy conducted by an ophthalmologist has high specificity but a low sensitivity of 34–50% in detecting early diabetic retinopathy [22].

There are two forms of diabetic retinopathy. Nonproliferative diabetic retinopathy (NPDR) consists of microaneurysms, dot "hemorrhages," cotton wool spots, and hard exudates. Dot hemorrhages are microaneurysms seen in cross section.

Proliferative diabetic retinopathy (PDR) has neovascularization, scar tissue formation with or without vitreous hemorrhage, and retinal detachment as manifestations [23].

Pathophysiology
Multiple mechanisms are involved in the pathogenesis of diabetic retinopathy; a few of them will be reviewed here.

Polyol Pathway The deleterious effect of sorbitol in retinal cells is due to the impermeability of the retinal cellular membranes to sorbitol. High concentrations of sorbitol accumulate and cause significant osmotic damage to the retina [24] (Fig. 4.1).

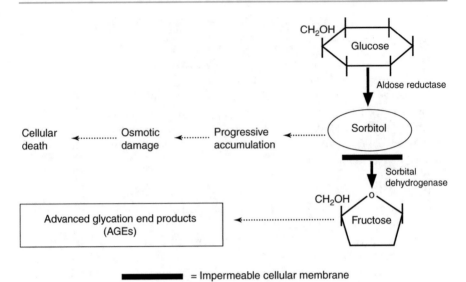

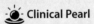

Fig. 4.1 Schematic representation of the polyol pathway and effects of glucotoxicity. The polyol pathway is involved in the metabolic handling of excess glucose. Glucose is reduced to sorbitol by aldose reductase, which is then converted into fructose by the sorbitol dehydrogenase enzyme [24]. Glucotoxicity results in an increased production of the intermediate product, sorbitol, which causes osmotic damage in involved tissues resulting not only in retinopathy but neuropathy and nephropathy as well. Breakdown products of fructose cause further damage to the retina by being converted to advanced glycation end products [25]. (Redrawn and modified from Tarr et al. [24])

Advanced Glycation End Products (AGEs)   AGEs are not synonymous with diabetes only; they indeed occur in normal human physiology. The difference in diabetes mellitus happens to be the accelerated rate of accumulation of these deleterious factors [26].

AGEs bind to their cognate receptor, i.e., receptor for AGE (RAGE). RAGE receptors are present in multiple tissues, including but not limited to the vasculature, renal, hepatic, central nervous system, and smooth muscle [26].

RAGE is abundant in retinal tissue; thus, AGE-to-RAGE binding initiates an inflammatory cascade, which results in neurovascular damage and eventual development of diabetic retinopathy [27] (Table 4.3).

☀ Clinical Pearl

Accumulation of sorbitol in the lens of the eye results in significant osmotic changes that predispose the diabetic eye to both refractive errors and cataract formation [30].

Table 4.3 Reasons for the fundoscopic findings of diabetic retinopathy

Fundoscopic finding (category of retinopathy)	Remarks
Microaneurysms of retinal capillaries (NPDR)	Chronic hyperglycemia-induced apoptosis of capillary pericytes (required to ensure the structural integrity of capillaries) [28]
Hard exudates (NPDR)	Increased capillary permeability and extrusion of proteinaceous exudate (hard exudates) [23]
Dot-and-blot hemorrhages (NPDR)	Extrusion of red blood cells out of capillaries results in areas of hemorrhage with either distinct (dot) or indistinct (blot) margins [28]
Neovascularization (PDR)	Progressive injury to retinal vessels causes ischemia and secondary formation of new vessels (hypoxia causes the release of proangiogenic growth factors) [29]
Retinal detachment (PDR)	Friable new vessels lead to vitreous hemorrhage and formation of fibrous tissue. The contraction of fibrotic bands causes retinal detachment [29]
Macular edema (PDR)	Hemorrhagic fluid leaking into the macula [23]

NPDR nonproliferative diabetic retinopathy, *PDR* proliferative diabetic retinopathy
Adapted from Corcóstegui [23], Wang [28], and Duh [29]

4.1.7   The Diabetic Foot

Clinical Features
The dreaded diabetic foot, a complication of uncontrolled diabetes, predisposes patients to foot ulcers, with an estimated lifetime risk of 25% [31]. There are two reported variants of the diabetic foot in the literature; these include the neuropathic and neuroischemic subtypes. As the name implies, the neuropathic foot has neuropathy as the underlying microvascular complication. The neuroischemic foot has neuropathy and vasculopathy coexisting in the same foot [32].

Pathophysiology
1. The polyol pathway, which was previously reviewed in the pathogenesis of diabetic retinopathy, mediates diabetic neuropathy (see Sect. 4.1.6). Accumulation of sorbitol and fructose impairs conductive neuronal function by reducing the synthesis of myoinositol [31]. There is evidence that exogenous myoinositol supplementation in patients with diabetic peripheral neuropathy significantly improves symptom scores, sensory and motor nerve conduction velocity, and neuronal action potential amplitude [33]. This is because myoinositol plays a permissive role in nerve conduction by upregulating neuronal sodium-potassium ATPase activity [34].
2. Depletion of folic acid, B6, and B12 also contributes to diabetic neuropathy, possibly through an increase in homocysteine. Metformin accelerates clearance of both folic acid and B12 and paradoxically increases the prevalence of neuropathy despite improved glycemic control [35–37]. There is evidence from both preclinical and clinical studies in subjects with diabetic peripheral neuropathy (DPN) which point not only to significantly improved neuropathy symptom

scores but also considerably improved nerve fiber density after a trial of a proprietary combination of L-methylfolate, B6, and B12 [38, 39].

3. Motor neuropathy leads to anatomic defects of the foot (Charcot's foot) [31].
4. Autonomic neuropathy impairs the function of sweat glands, leading to xerosis, which predisposes the involved foot to skin breaks [31].
5. Sensory neuropathy causes an insensate foot and predisposes the involved foot to unrecognized injury [31].

    Vasculopathy occurs due to the harmful effects of reactive oxygen species (ROS) on the vasculature. Nicotinamide adenine dinucleotide phosphate (NADPH) is depleted in the polyol pathway; this leads to the accumulation of reactive oxygen species (ROS) since NADPH is unable to play its "scavenger role" [31].

6. NADPH is involved in the formation of nitric oxide, a potent vasodilator. NADPH depletion via the polyol pathway results in reduced levels of nitric oxide [31].

 Pathophysiology Pearl

Pathophysiologic Basis of Metformin-Induced Vitamin B12 Deficiency

1. Altered bowel transit time leading to small intestinal bacterial overgrowth and impaired absorption of vitamin B12 [40].
2. Metformin directly inhibits calcium-dependent vitamin B12-intrinsic factor transfer at the terminal ileum [40].

 Clinical Pearl

The Best Screening Test for Diabetic Peripheral Neuropathy (DPN)

    Loss of vibratory sensation (detected with a 128 Hz tuning fork) is the first objective clinical sign in DPN. It can provide a more sensitive quantitative assessment of DPN even in patients with apparently normal standard 10 g monofilament test results [41].

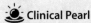 **Questions You Might Be Asked on Clinical Rounds**

Briefly describe the mechanisms involved in the development of insulin resistance in T2DM patients?

1. There is a reversible defect in tyrosine kinase activity of insulin receptors present in the liver, adipose tissue, and muscle. This post-receptor signaling defect leads to reduced metabolic effects of insulin, including a decrease in glycogen synthase activity, an increase in hepatic gluconeogenesis, and a reduction in lipolysis [42].

2. Reduced glucose transporter 4 (GLUT-4) expression in skeletal muscle and adipose tissue accounts for hyperglycemia in insulin resistance [43–45].
3. Continuous exposure to insulin in the setting of endogenous hyperinsulinemia, in contrast to physiologic pulsatile insulin exposure, has been shown to cause progressive downregulation of peripheral insulin receptors [46].

What are the causes of insulin resistance?
There are three types of insulin resistance.

• Type A insulin resistance occurs as a result of impaired function of the insulin receptor due to mutations in the insulin receptor gene [47].
• Type B insulin resistance is due to antibodies directed against the insulin receptor [48].
• Type C insulin resistance is due to post-insulin receptor dysfunction (impaired downstream action of insulin) [49].

Intrinsic defects occur as a result of a defect in the insulin receptor gene, which impairs its normal physiologic function. Extrinsic defects are due to circulating factors, e.g., hormones and inflammatory cytokines, which interfere with insulin to insulin receptor binding [50] (Table 4.4).

Table 4.4   Causes of insulin resistance by the underlying mechanism

Intrinsic defects	Extrinsic defects
Leprechaunism (Donohue syndrome) [47, 51][a]	Pregnancy (physiologic cause) [52]
Rabson-Mendenhall syndrome [47, 53][a]	Infection and starvation (stress-related conditions) [54]
Congenital generalized lipodystrophy [55, 56]	Glucagonoma [57, 58], thyroid dysfunction [59], pheochromocytoma [57, 60], acromegaly(endocrinopathies) [61]
Familial partial lipodystrophy (Dunnigan variant) [62]	Type B insulin resistance due to insulin receptor inhibitory antibodies [48, 63]

[a]Type A insulin resistance (hyperandrogenism, insulin resistance, and acanthosis nigricans)
Adapted from Refs. [47, 48, 51–58, 60–62]

4.2   Rabson-Mendenhall Syndrome
(Type A Insulin Resistance)

4.2.1   Acanthosis Nigricans

Clinical Features
Acanthosis nigricans is a dermatologic manifestation of type A insulin resistance syndromes [64–66]. The clinical features of acanthosis nigricans have been previously described (see Sect. 4.1.1).

Pathophysiology
The pathophysiologic basis for acanthosis nigricans due to endogenous hyperinsulinemia has been previously described (see Sect. 4.1.1).

Rabson-Mendenhall syndrome is a Type A insulin resistance syndrome that occurs as a result of mutation of the insulin receptor gene. Intracellular signaling pathways, including tyrosine phosphorylation and other downstream processes, become defective, leading to significant impairment in insulin action in target organs [65, 66].

Persistent hyperinsulinemia accounts for some of the physical manifestations of RMS, including hypertrichosis and xerosis [67] (Table 4.5).

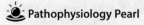 Pathophysiology Pearl
Mechanism of Insulin Secretion (Fig. 4.2)

Table 4.5 Other physical manifestations of RMS and their underlying pathophysiologic mechanisms

Physical finding(s)	Pathophysiology
Organomegaly (phallic enlargement, clitoromegaly, and nephromegaly) [68]	IGF-1, which is a growth factor, shares structural homology with insulin. Hyperinsulinemia accounts for organomegaly due to the effects of insulin on the IGF-1 receptor [69]
Hypertrichosis and xerosis [68]	Insulin binding to IGF-1 receptors in the integument [68]

Adapted from Sinnarajah [68] and Chong [69]

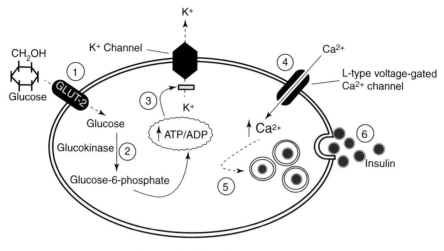

Pancreatic beta cell

Fig. 4.2 Mechanism of insulin secretion in the postprandial state. In the fasting (basal) state, the pancreatic cell membrane remains hyperpolarized, thus limiting insulin secretion. After a meal, glucose is actively transported into the cytoplasm of the pancreatic beta-cell by glucose transporter 2 (GLUT-2) (step 1) [70, 71]. Glucose goes through an initial phosphorylation step, which is facilitated by glucokinase (glycolysis) (step 2). Glycolysis generates a high concentration of intracytoplasmic ATP, which then inhibits ATP-sensitive potassium channels on the plasma membrane (step 3) [72, 73]. Impaired potassium conductance leads to depolarization of the plasma membrane and subsequent activation of voltage-gated calcium channels [74]. These activated calcium channels funnel calcium into the cytoplasm of the pancreatic beta-cell (step 4), where they mediate the release of preformed insulin from the secretory granules through a process of exocytosis (steps 5 and 6) [75]. (Redrawn and modified from Fu et al. [70])

💡 Questions You Might Be Asked on Clinical Rounds

What are the objective methods for assessing insulin resistance?

Assessment of insulin resistance is limited by the lack of a single measure, which is both accurate and applicable in routine clinical practice.

- The hyperinsulinemic-euglycemic glucose clamp
- Fasting insulin levels
- Glucose to insulin ratio
- The homeostatic model assessment of insulin resistance (HOMA-IR)
- QUICKI (an equation dependent on fasting blood glucose and insulin levels)
- Frequently sampled intravenous glucose tolerance tests

There are other measures of insulin resistance, which are beyond the scope of this book. The gold standard of measuring insulin resistance is the hyperinsulinemic-euglycemic clamp. It is, however, labor-intensive and not applicable in practice [76].

Briefly discuss the phases of insulin secretion in normal physiology
Basal Insulin Physiology

In the fasting (basal) state, insulin is released through an interplay of rapid 5 to 15 minute pulses of insulin release and much longer and slower ultradian oscillations, which last approximately 80–180 minutes [77].

Postprandial Insulin Physiology

The first phase of insulin secretion involves the release of preformed insulin from storage vesicles. This initial step is vital in reducing hepatic glucose output after a meal.

The second phase involves a more gradual process that requires the synthesis of new insulin. This phase mediates glucose uptake in skeletal muscle and adipose tissue [78].

4.3   Glucagonoma

4.3.1   Necrolytic Migratory Erythema

Clinical Features

Necrolytic migratory erythema (NME) is a pathognomonic dermatosis of the glucagonoma syndrome. NME is the presenting feature of the glucagonoma syndrome in up to 70% of patients [79, 80]. Skin lesions are annular, crusted, erythematous plaques distributed over mainly intertriginous areas, but may be seen on the extremities and trunk as well [79]. The lesions may be easily misdiagnosed as other causes of dermatoses, leading to delayed diagnosis in most patients [80, 81].

Pathophysiology

The mechanisms underlying the clinical manifestation of NME are yet to be clarified. These are, however, some proposed mechanisms.

1. Glucagon, being a counterregulatory hormone in glucose metabolism, promotes gluconeogenesis, which results in the depletion of protein in the epidermal layer of the skin. This promotes necrolysis in the epidermis [79].
2. Vitamin B, zinc [82], and fatty acid deficiencies are possible reasons for the similarity between NME and other cutaneous dermatoses associated with these deficiency states. Reduction in levels of glucagon either with tumor resection or somatostatin analog therapy results in prompt resolution of NME [79].

Table 4.6 Clinical features and underlying mechanisms of some manifestations of the glucagonoma syndrome

Clinical feature	Mechanism(s)
Weight loss	Glucagon acts on glucagon-like peptide-1 (GLP-1) receptors in central satiety centers (anorexigenic pathway) to facilitate weight loss [83] Stimulates energy expenditure by activating thermogenesis in brown adipose tissue [83]
Cardiomyopathy and heart failure	Glucagon binding to its G-protein-coupled receptor increases intracellular cyclic AMP, which activates protein kinase A (PKA). PKA mediates the phosphorylation of L-type calcium channels of the cardiomyocyte sarcolemma. This results in an influx of calcium, which promotes increased myocardial contraction. Prolonged activation of the sarcoplasmic reticulum leads to calcium leak, accentuated myocardial contractility, and eventual cardiac remodeling [84, 85]

Adapted from Albrechtsen [83], Zhang [84], and Demir [85]

 Questions You Might Be Asked on Clinical Rounds

What are some other clinical features of the glucagonoma syndrome? (Table 4.6)

What is pseudoglucagonoma syndrome, and how can it be differentiated from the classic glucagonoma syndrome?
Pseudoglucagonoma syndrome can present with clinical features of a glucagonoma in the absence of an alpha-cell tumor of the pancreas. Patients may have either elevated or normal glucagon levels and, in some cases, present with the characteristic NME rash. Malignancies, chronic liver disease, pancreatitis, and non-tropical sprue are known causes of pseudoglucagonoma syndrome [86].

4.4 Carcinoid Syndrome

4.4.1 Cutaneous Flushing

Clinical Features
Cutaneous flushing has a mean prevalence of 78%, based on cumulative evidence from case series [87]. It classically involves the face, neck, and upper chest [88] and is usually triggered by amine-rich foods, pharmacologic agents, or emotional stress [89].

Repeated episodes of flushing which tend to be transient (lasting 10–30 minutes) are characteristic of midgut carcinoids. A longer-lasting duration of flushing (up to several hours) is more characteristic of foregut carcinoids [88].

Pathophysiology

Cutaneous flushing is caused by various vasoactive mediators, including, but not limited to, *histamine, substance P*, and *prostaglandins*. Interestingly, serotonin blockers do not improve the pathognomonic flushing associated with carcinoid syndrome. This rules out serotonin as the bioactive hormone involved in the cutaneous flushing of carcinoid syndrome (CS) [87].

The duration of flushing is dependent on the venous drainage of the involved organ. Foregut NETs bypass initial hepatic metabolism; as such, the vasoactive amines persist longer in circulation, resulting in a more prolonged period of flushing. Midgut carcinoids, on the other hand, tend to cause flushing in the setting of hepatic metastases [88].

> **Associated Endocrinopathies/Conditions That Can Present with Flushing**
> Pheochromocytomas, Cushing's syndrome, medullary thyroid cancer, rosacea, and mastocytosis [89]

>  **Clinical Pearl**
> Nature of Flushing and Underlying Etiology
> If flushing is dry (i.e., no concomitant hyperhidrosis), then it is of neuroendocrine etiology. If it is wet (i.e., associated hyperhidrosis), then it is most likely of another etiology other than a neuroendocrine origin (e.g., menopause or anxiety disorder) [88].

4.4.2 Diarrhea

Clinical Features

There is a variable reported prevalence of diarrhea, ranging from 58% to 100% with a mean of 78% in multiple case series [87]. Diarrhea tends to be secretory and, as such, persists even when the patient is fasting. This should be contrasted from non-secretory diarrhea, which improves during a fast and is usually of other etiology [88].

Pathophysiology

Serotonin is believed to be the active peptide mediating diarrhea in patients with the carcinoid syndrome. Serotonin promotes an increased secretion of intestinal fluid and ions in the small intestine, which exceeds the bowels' net absorptive capacity, resulting in secretory diarrhea. Telotristat ethyl inhibits the rate-limiting step of serotonin synthesis by impairing the function of TH-1 (see Fig. 4.3) [87, 92]. Amelioration of the symptoms of diarrhea with this TH-1 inhibitor confirms the role of serotonin in the diarrhea of carcinoid syndrome [87].

> 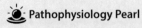 **Pathophysiology Pearl**
> Neuroendocrine Tumor Cellular Model

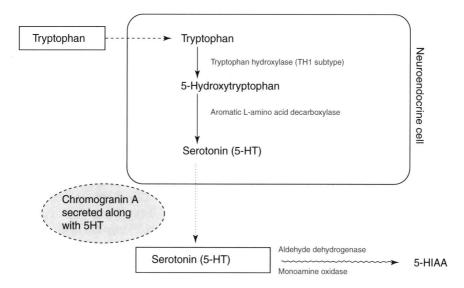

Fig. 4.3 Schematic diagram of the biosynthesis of serotonin. Tryptophan hydroxylase 1 (TH-1) is the rate-limiting enzyme in serotonin synthesis by neuroendocrine tumors and is expressed in various tissues, including the gastrointestinal tract, spleen, thymus, and pineal glands [90]. Tryptophan is initially transported into the neuroendocrine cell (dashed arrow). Tryptophan is then converted into 5-hydroxytryptophan by tryptophan hydroxylase-1 enzyme [87, 91]. The conversion of 5-hydroxytryptophan into serotonin (5-hydroxytryptamine, 5-HT) occurs in an intermediate decarboxylation step, which requires aromatic L-acid decarboxylase. 5-HT is packaged along with chromogranin A (a neuroendocrine tumor marker) and is then released into circulation (dotted arrow). 5-HT undergoes metabolism via various enzymatic conversion steps, which result in the formation of 5-Hydroxyindoleacetic acid (5-HIAA) (an inactive metabolite) (wavy arrow) [87, 91]. (Redrawn and modified from Frazer and Hensler [91])

4.4.3 Bronchospasm

Clinical Features
Patients present with audible wheezing and confirmatory rhonchi on auscultation. The prevalence of asthma-like features is, however, less frequent when compared to diarrhea and cutaneous flushing. The reported prevalence rate based on large case series is about 3–18% [87]. Carcinoid syndrome can be misdiagnosed as asthma, and treatment with standard anti-bronchospastic therapies can result in the worsening of symptoms [93].

Pathophysiology
- Bioactive amines such as serotonin mediate bronchospasm.
- Bronchospasm could also be due to central airway obstruction due to the endobronchial location of pulmonary carcinoids [94].

4.4.4   Cardiac Valvular Lesions

Clinical Features
Carcinoid heart disease (CHD) has a prevalence rate ranging from 11% to 70% [87]. Patients can present with right-sided murmurs (tricuspid and pulmonary valves), peripheral edema, ascites, and other signs of right-sided heart failure [95].

Pathophysiology
The most cited pathophysiologic mechanism happens to be a serotoninergic-mediated process. Binding of serotonin to ubiquitous 5-Hydroxytryptamine receptor 2B (5-HT2B) receptors in the heart explains the clinical manifestations of CHD [87].

Serotonin and other vasoactive amines stimulate 5-HT2B receptors present on the surface of myofibroblasts. This leads to fibrosis and deposition of myxomatous substances in the endocardium. Again, telotristat, a novel tryptophan hydroxylase enzyme inhibitor, retarded CHD in two patients enrolled in the landmark TELESTAR (Telotristat Etiprate for Somatostatin Analogue Not Adequately Controlled Carcinoid Syndrome) phase III trial, further affirming the role of serotonin in this condition [87].

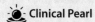 **Clinical Pearl**

Carcinoid Heart Disease
Carcinoid heart disease tends to involve the right side of the heart more often than the left, due to the inactivation of serotonin in the lung. This leads to the sparing of the left side of the heart from this vasoactive amine [95].

Indeed, left-sided cardiac involvement occurs in patients' with coexisting intracardiac shunts since serotonin can bypass "pulmonary inactivation" to some degree [87].

Left-sided carcinoid heart disease is also common in the context of a high burden of disease (overwhelms inactivation systems) or carcinoids located in the bronchopulmonary tree [95].

4.4.5   Other Cutaneous Manifestations (Pellagra)

Clinical Features
Pellagra is described in many medical texts as a syndrome composed of dermatitis, diarrhea, dementia, and death. The mnemonic "4Ds," is well-known by many medical professionals. It is a photosensitive rash that tends to involve sun-exposed areas such as the face, neck, and forearms. The rash is characteristically hyperpigmented and scaly [96].

Pathophysiology

Niacin deficiency occurs as a result of significant shunting of tryptophan from niacin synthesis to serotonin synthesis. This is even more profound in patients with a sizeable metastatic carcinoid tumor burden [97].

Other cutaneous manifestations of carcinoid syndrome include scleroderma [98], vitiligo, psoriasis, pityriasis versicolor, and Campbell de Morgan spots (cherry red angiomas). The exact mechanism is unknown but may be due to the cutaneous effects of a host of vasoactive substances, including prostaglandins, serotonin, histamine, and bradykinin [99].

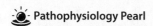 **Pathophysiology Pearl**

Achlorhydria-Induced Gastric Carcinoids
   How does achlorhydria result in the formation of gastric carcinoids? (Fig. 4.4)

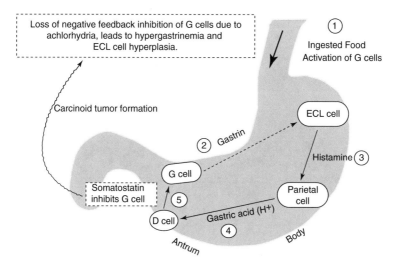

Fig. 4.4 Schematic diagram of achlorhydria-induced gastric carcinoid formation. Ingestion of food leads to the activation of the G cells of the stomach (step 1). The G cells present in the gastric antrum release gastrin after the ingestion of food (step 2). Gastrin, in turn, binds to CCK receptors present on gastric enterochromaffin-like (ECL) cells (dashed arrow), inducing the release of histamine (step 3). Histamine, in turn, binds to H2 receptors on the cell membranes of gastric parietal cells inducing the release of hydrochloric acid (step 4). The acidic milieu of the gut is critical in stimulating the release of somatostatin by the delta-cells of the pancreas (step 5). Somatostatin is critical in providing negative feedback inhibition of gastrin release from the G cells. In the setting of achlorhydria as might occur in pernicious anemia (antiparietal cell receptor antibody-mediated anemia), this negative feedback loop involving somatostatin is impaired. This results in the uncontrolled release of gastrin from the G cells [100]. Gastrin, apart from stimulating increased histamine production from gastric ECL cells, also leads to their unchecked proliferation (hyperplasia) (dashed boxes). This uncontrolled proliferation can lead to gain-of-function mutations and eventual tumorigenesis (carcinoid formation) [101]. (Based on Nikou et al. [100])

Questions You Might Be Asked on Clinical Rounds

Which neuroendocrine tumors (NETs) can present with carcinoid syndrome (CS) in the absence of hepatic metastases?

CS has traditionally been assumed only to occur when bioactive neuropeptides bypass hepatic inactivation resulting in exposure of these hormones to the systemic circulation in patients with gastrointestinal NETs. It is worthy to note that NETs originating from the ovary, testis, and pancreas can present with CS in the absence of hepatic metastasis [87].

Define carcinoids and the carcinoid syndrome

Carcinoids/Carcinoid Tumors

These are tumors of cells derived from *enterochromaffin cells* [102]. The clinical features of carcinoid tumors or carcinoids were described in 1907 by Oberndorfer. He reported the following features as being pathognomonic of carcinoids, i.e., small, undifferentiated, well-defined borders, and slow growing [103].

Carcinoid tumors are now appreciated as tumors with a malignant predisposition and were redefined in the year 2000 by the World Health Organization as *neuroendocrine tumors* (NETs) [104]. Older references to NETs include *carcinoids*, *APUDoma*, *argentaffinoma*, and *argyrophilic cell carcinoma* [104].

Carcinoid Syndrome

Carcinoid syndrome occurs when carcinoid tumors release various peptides and vasoactive amines directly into the systemic circulation, especially in the setting of pulmonary or hepatic metastases [102].

4.5   VIPoma

4.5.1   Dehydration Due to Extrarenal Losses

Clinical Features

Secretory diarrhea is a component of WDHA (watery diarrhea, hypokalemia, hypochlorhydria or achlorhydria) syndrome, a common tetrad observed in patients with VIPomas. Due to the significant amount of gastrointestinal fluid and electrolyte losses, patients can develop dehydration with resultant hypotension and acute kidney injury [105].

Pathophysiology

Vasoactive intestinal peptide (VIP) potentiates the effect of cyclic adenosine monophosphate (cAMP) at the level of the intestinal epithelium [106] and through various intracellular processes results in increased gut motility, increased gastrointestinal fluid output, and electrolyte losses [105, 107].

Clinical Pearl

NET differentials of chronic diarrhea:

- VIPoma should always be considered as a pancreatic neuroendocrine manifestation of MEN-1 [108].
- Chronic diarrhea also occurs in Zollinger-Ellison syndrome (gastrinoma) due to suboptimal intestinal absorption of excessive gastric acid output. In a study involving over 2000 subjects at the National Institutes of Health (NIH), fasting serum gastrin levels had a positive correlation with diarrhea as a presenting feature of Zollinger-Ellison syndrome [109].

Questions You Might Be Asked on Clinical Rounds

What are the biochemical abnormalities in patients with VIPomas? (Table 4.7)
What is vasoactive intestinal peptide (VIP)?

- It is a polypeptide with intrinsic adenylate cyclase-activating properties [110].
- It is expressed in various tissues, including the central nervous system and gastrointestinal, respiratory, and genital tracts [110].

Effects of VIP

- Gastrointestinal smooth muscle contraction
- Vasodilation
- Increased gastrointestinal and pancreatic secretions [111]

Briefly discuss the other neuroendocrine tumors (NETs) of the pancreas apart from VIPomas and glucagonomas

The islets of Langerhans in the pancreas are composed of various cell types (see Table 4.8). There are several reported pathogenesis models for NETs [125] well beyond the scope of this book; nonetheless, pancreatic NETs in simple terms are derived from pancreatic ductal stem cells capable of differentiating into the various pancreatic cell subtypes [126, 127].

Table 4.7 Pathophysiologic basis for biochemical abnormalities in VIPoma syndromes

Biochemical abnormality	Mechanisms
Hypokalemia	1. Gastrointestinal losses due to diarrhea [105]
	2. Secondary hyperaldosteronism due to volume contraction [105]
	3. Loss of potassium from enterocytes [105]
Hypercalcemia	Hyperparathyroidism due to MEN1 [105]
Non-anion gap metabolic acidosis	Diarrhea [105]

Adapted from Abu-Zaid et al. [105]

Table 4.8 Pancreatic islet cells and their corresponding hormones

Islet cell (frequency)	Hormone produced	Effects(s)
Beta-cells (50–70%)	Insulin and amylin	Insulin increases peripheral glucose uptake and reduces hepatic gluconeogenesis and glycogenolysis [112, 113] Amylin slows gastric emptying and stimulates satiety [114]
Alpha-cells (20–30%)	Glucagon	Stimulates hepatic gluconeogenesis and glycogenolysis. Stimulates hepatic ketogenesis during a prolonged fast [115, 116]
Delta-cells (10%)	Somatostatin	Inhibits the secretion of insulin, glucagon, and PP [112]
PP cells (2%)	Pancreatic polypeptide	Inhibition of glucagon secretion and acts as a satiety hormone [112]
Epsilon cells (1%)	Ghrelin	Inhibits insulin release after a glucose load. Stimulates GH secretion and is also called the "hunger hormone" [117]
G cells (absent)	Gastrin	Pancreatic gastrin producing cells are present during embryonic development but undergo involution in adults. Re-expression of gastrin can, however, occur in the setting of pancreatic neuroendocrine tumorigenesis (Zollinger-Ellison Syndrome) [118]. See hypergastrinemia effects in Table 4.9
EC cells (rare)	Serotonin	Classic features of carcinoid syndrome [123, 124]

GH growth hormone, *EC* enterochromaffin cells, *PP* pancreatic polypeptide
Adapted from Refs. [112–118, 123, 124]

Table 4.9 Other neuroendocrine tumors of the pancreas

NET	Clinical feature(s) (pathophysiology)
Insulinoma	Whipple's triad (hyperinsulinemia-induced reduction in glycogenolysis and gluconeogenesis. Also, insulin promotes increased glucose uptake in peripheral tissues) [119] Weight gain (anabolic effects of insulin) [119]
Gastrinoma	Multiple peptic ulcers (hypergastrinemia-mediated increased gastric acid output) [120] Secretory diarrhea (increased gastric acid output reduces bowel transit time) [120]
PPoma (pancreatic polypeptide tumor)	Weight loss and abdominal discomfort (stimulation of gastrointestinal enzyme secretions) [121]
Somatostatinoma	Complicated gallstones (somatostatin reduces gallbladder contractility and secretions leading to sludging and stone formation) [122] Steatorrhea (impaired release of bilious fluid from the gallbladder) [122] Hyperglycemia complications (inhibition of insulin secretion) [122]

Adapted from Refs. [119–122]

The other NETs of pancreatic origin include gastrinoma, insulinoma, somatostatinoma, and PPoma. See Table 4.9 for the pathophysiologic basis of the clinical features of these NETs.

References

1. Karadağ AS, You Y, Danarti R, Al-Khuzaei S, Chen W. Acanthosis nigricans and the metabolic syndrome. Clin Dermatol. 2018;36:48–53.
2. Bustan RS, Wasim D, Yderstræde KB, Bygum A. Specific skin signs as a cutaneous marker of diabetes mellitus and the prediabetic state – a systematic review. Dan Med J. 2017;64:A5316.
3. Duff M, Demidova O, Blackburn S, Shubrook J. Cutaneous manifestations of diabetes mellitus. Clin Diabetes. 2015;33:40–8.
4. Mistry BD, Alavi A, Ali S, Mistry N. A systematic review of the relationship between glycemic control and necrobiosis lipoidica diabeticorum in patients with diabetes mellitus. Int J Dermatol. 2017;56:1319–27.
5. Gentile S, Strollo F, Ceriello A. Lipodystrophy in insulin-treated subjects and other injection-site skin reactions: are we sure everything is clear? Diabetes Ther. 2016;7:401–9.
6. Heinemann L. Insulin absorption from lipodystrophic areas: a (neglected) source of trouble for insulin therapy? J Diabetes Sci Technol. 2010;4:750–3.
7. Deng N, Zhang X, Zhao F, Wang Y, He H. Prevalence of lipohypertrophy in insulin-treated diabetes patients: a systematic review and meta-analysis. J Diabetes Investig. 2018;9:536–43.
8. Thornsberry LA, English JC. Etiology, diagnosis, and therapeutic management of granuloma annulare: an update. Am J Clin Dermatol. 2013;14:279–90.
9. Atkinson MA, Eisenbarth GS, Michels AW. Type 1 diabetes. Lancet. 2014;383:69–82.
10. DeFronzo RA. Pathogenesis of type 2 diabetes mellitus. Med Clin N Am. 2004;88:787–835.
11. Plows JF, Stanley JL, Baker PN, Reynolds CM, Vickers MH. The pathophysiology of gestational diabetes mellitus. Int J Mol Sci. 2018;19(11):3342. https://doi.org/10.3390/ijms19113342.
12. Kayani K, Mohammed R, Mohiaddin H. Cystic fibrosis-related diabetes. Front Endocrinol. 2018;9:20.
13. Shivaswamy V, Boerner B, Larsen J. Post-transplant diabetes mellitus: causes, treatment, and impact on outcomes. Endocr Rev. 2016;37:37–61.
14. American Diabetes Association. 2. Classification and diagnosis of diabetes: standards of medical care in diabetes-2020. Diabetes Care. 2020;43:S14–31.
15. Hart PA, Bellin MD, Andersen DK, et al. Type 3c (pancreatogenic) diabetes mellitus secondary to chronic pancreatitis and pancreatic cancer. Lancet Gastroenterol Hepatol. 2016;1:226–37.
16. Fajans SS, Bell GI. MODY: history, genetics, pathophysiology, and clinical decision making. Diabetes Care. 2011;34:1878–84.
17. Weinreich SS, Bosma A, Henneman L, Rigter T, Spruijt CM, Grimbergen AJ, et al. A decade of molecular genetic testing for MODY: a retrospective study of utilization in The Netherlands. Eur J Hum Genet. 2015;23:29–33.
18. Carlsson S. Etiology and pathogenesis of latent autoimmune diabetes in adults (LADA) compared to type 2 diabetes. Front Physiol. 2019;10:320.
19. Spellberg B, Edwards J, Ibrahim A. Novel perspectives on mucormycosis: pathophysiology, presentation, and management. Clin Microbiol Rev. 2005;18:556–69.
20. Vijayabala GS, Annigeri RG, Sudarshan R. Mucormycosis in a diabetic ketoacidosis patient. Asian Pac J Trop Biomed. 2013;3:830–3.
21. Schulz C, Moore J, Hassan D, Tamsett E, Smith CF. Addressing the 'forgotten art of "fundoscopy"': evaluation of a novel teaching ophthalmoscope'. Eye (Lond). 2016;30:375–84.
22. Singh R, Ramasamy K, Abraham C, Gupta V, Gupta A. Diabetic retinopathy: an update. Indian J Ophthalmol. 2008;56:179–88.
23. Corcóstegui B, Durán S, González-Albarrán MO, Hernández C, Ruiz-Moreno JM, Salvador J, et al. Update on diagnosis and treatment of diabetic retinopathy: a consensus guideline of the Working Group of Ocular Health (Spanish Society of Diabetes and Spanish Vitreous and Retina Society). J Ophthalmol. 2017;2017:8234186. https://doi.org/10.1155/2017/8234186.
24. Tarr JM, Kaul K, Chopra M, Kohner EM, Chibber R. Pathophysiology of diabetic retinopathy. ISRN Ophthalmol. 2013;2013:343560. https://doi.org/10.1155/2013/343560.

25. Yan L. Redox imbalance stress in diabetes mellitus: role of the polyol pathway. Animal Model Exp Med. 2018;1:7–13.
26. Stitt AW. AGEs and diabetic retinopathy. Invest Ophthalmol Vis Sci. 2010;51:4867–74.
27. Zong H, Ward M, Stitt AW. AGEs, RAGE, and diabetic retinopathy. Curr Diab Rep. 2011;11:244–52.
28. Wang W, Lo ACY. Diabetic retinopathy: pathophysiology and treatments. Int J Mol Sci. 2018;19(6):1816. https://doi.org/10.3390/ijms19061816.
29. Duh EJ, Sun JK, Stitt AW. Diabetic retinopathy: current understanding, mechanisms, and treatment strategies. JCI Insight. 2017;2(14):e93751. https://doi.org/10.1172/jci.insight.93751.
30. Pollreisz A, Schmidt-Erfurth U. Diabetic cataract—pathogenesis. J Ophthalmol. 2010;2010:608751. https://doi.org/10.1155/2010/608751.
31. Clayton W, Elasy TA. A review of the pathophysiology, classification, and treatment of foot ulcers in diabetic patients. Clin Diabetes. 2009;27:52–8.
32. Pendsey SP. Understanding diabetic foot. Int J Diabetes Dev Ctries. 2010;30:75–9.
33. Clements RS. Dietary myo-inositol and diabetic neuropathy. Adv Exp Med Biol. 1979;119:287–94.
34. Zychowska M, Rojewska E, Przewlocka B, Mika J. Mechanisms and pharmacology of diabetic neuropathy – experimental and clinical studies. Pharmacol Rep. 2013;65:1601–10.
35. Xu L, Huang Z, He X, Wan X, Fang D, Li Y. Adverse effect of metformin therapy on serum vitamin B12 and folate: short-term treatment causes disadvantages? Med Hypotheses. 2013;81:149–51.
36. Esmaeilzadeh S, Gholinezhad-Chari M, Ghadimi R. The effect of metformin treatment on the serum levels of homocysteine, folic acid, and vitamin B12 in patients with polycystic ovary syndrome. J Hum Reprod Sci. 2017;10:95.
37. Aroda VR, Edelstein SL, Goldberg RB, et al. Long-term metformin use and vitamin B12 deficiency in the diabetes prevention program outcomes study. J Clin Endocrinol Metab. 2016;101:1754–61.
38. Jayabalan B, Low LL. Vitamin B supplementation for diabetic peripheral neuropathy. Singap Med J. 2016;57:55–9.
39. Fonseca VA, Lavery LA, Thethi TK, Daoud Y, DeSouza C, Ovalle F, et al. Metanx in type 2 diabetes with peripheral neuropathy: a randomized trial. Am J Med. 2013;126:141–9.
40. Akinlade KS, Agbebaku SO, Rahamon SK, Balogun WO. Vitamin B12 levels in patients with type 2 diabetes mellitus on metformin. Ann Ib Postgrad Med. 2015;13:79–83.
41. Oyer DS, Saxon D, Shah A. Quantitative assessment of diabetic peripheral neuropathy with use of the clanging tuning fork test. Endocr Pract. 2007;13:5–10.
42. Petersen KF, Shulman GI. Etiology of insulin resistance. Am J Med. 2006;119:S10–6.
43. Leguisamo NM, Lehnen AM, Machado UF, Okamoto MM, Markoski MM, Pinto GH, et al. GLUT4 content decreases along with insulin resistance and high levels of inflammatory markers in rats with metabolic syndrome. Cardiovasc Diabetol. 2012;11:100.
44. Xu P-T, Song Z, Zhang W-C, Jiao B, Yu Z-B. Impaired translocation of GLUT4 results in insulin resistance of atrophic soleus muscle. Biomed Res Int. 2015;2015:291987. https://doi.org/10.1155/2015/291987.
45. Atkinson BJ, Griesel BA, King CD, Josey MA, Olson AL. Moderate GLUT4 overexpression improves insulin sensitivity and fasting triglyceridemia in high-fat diet–fed transgenic mice. Diabetes. 2013;62:2249–58.
46. Shanik MH, Xu Y, Škrha J, Dankner R, Zick Y, Roth J. Insulin resistance and hyperinsulinemia: is hyperinsulinemia the cart or the horse? Diabetes Care. 2008;31:S262–8.
47. Young J, Morbois-Trabut L, Couzinet B, et al. Type A insulin resistance syndrome revealing a novel lamin A mutation. Diabetes. 2005;54:1873–8.
48. Malek R, Chong AY, Lupsa BC, Lungu AO, Cochran EK, Soos MA, et al. Treatment of type B insulin resistance: a novel approach to reduce insulin receptor autoantibodies. J Clin Endocrinol Metab. 2010;95:3641–7.
49. Hong JH, Kim HJ, Park KS, Ku BJ. Paradigm shift in the management of type B insulin resistance. Ann Transl Med. 2018;6(suppl 2):S98. https://doi.org/10.21037/atm.2018.11.21.

50. Diamanti-Kandarakis E, Dunaif A. Insulin resistance and the polycystic ovary syndrome revisited: An update on mechanisms and implications. Endocr Rev. 2012;33:981–1030.
51. Nijim Y, Awni Y, Adawi A, Bowirrat A. Classic case report of donohue syndrome (Leprechaunism; OMIM *246200): the impact of consanguineous mating. Medicine (Baltimore). 2016;95:e2710.
52. Hodson K, Man CD, Smith FE, Thelwall PE, Cobelli C, Robson SC, et al. Mechanism of insulin resistance in normal pregnancy. Horm Metab Res. 2013;45:567–71.
53. Bathi RJ, Parveen S, Mutalik S, Rao R. Rabson-Mendenhall syndrome: two case reports and a brief review of the literature. Odontology. 2010;98:89–96.
54. Wilcox G. Insulin and insulin resistance. Clin Biochem Rev. 2005;26:19–39.
55. Jeninga EH, de Vroede M, Hamers N, Breur JMPJ, Verhoeven-Duif NM, Berger R, et al. A patient with congenital generalized Lipodystrophy due to a novel mutation in BSCL2: indications for secondary mitochondrial dysfunction. JIMD Rep. 2011;4:47–54.
56. Agarwal AK, Barnes RI, Garg A. Genetic basis of congenital generalized lipodystrophy. Int J Obes Relat Metab Disord. 2004;28:336–9.
57. Rogowicz-Frontczak A, Majchrzak A, Zozulińska-Ziółkiewicz D. Insulin resistance in endocrine disorders - treatment options. Endokrynol Pol. 2017;68:334–51.
58. Castro PG, de León AM, Trancón JG, Martínez PÁ, Álvarez Pérez JA, Fernández Fernández JC, et al. Glucagonoma syndrome: a case report. J Med Case Rep. 2011;5:402.
59. Brenta G. Why can insulin resistance be a natural consequence of thyroid dysfunction? J Thyroid Res. 2011;2011:9. https://doi.org/10.4061/2011/152850.
60. Komada H, Hirota Y, So A, Nakamura T, Okuno Y, Fukuoka H, et al. Insulin secretion and insulin sensitivity before and after surgical treatment of pheochromocytoma or paraganglioma. J Clin Endocrinol Metab. 2017;102:3400–5.
61. Olarescu NC, Bollerslev J. The impact of adipose tissue on insulin resistance in acromegaly. Trends Endocrinol Metab. 2016;27:226–37.
62. Belo SPM, Magalhães ÂC, Freitas P, Carvalho DM. Familial partial lipodystrophy, Dunnigan variety – challenges for patient care during pregnancy: a case report. BMC Res Notes. 2015;8:140.
63. Bourron O, Vigouroux C, Halbron M, Touati EB, Capel E, Caron-Debarle M, et al. Association of type B Insulin resistance and type 1 diabetes resulting in ketoacidosis. Diabetes Care. 2012;35:e4.
64. Chen X, Wang H, Wu B, Dong X, Liu B, Chen H, et al. One novel 2.43Kb deletion and one single nucleotide mutation of the INSR gene in a Chinese neonate with Rabson-Mendenhall syndrome. J Clin Res Pediatr Endocrinol. 2018;10:183–7.
65. Moore MM, Bailey AM, Flannery AH, Baum RA. Treatment of diabetic ketoacidosis with intravenous U-500 insulin in a patient with Rabson-Mendenhall syndrome: a case report. J Pharm Pract. 2017;30:468–75.
66. Ben Abdelaziz R, Ben Chehida A, Azzouz H, Boudabbous H, Lascols O, Ben Turkia H, et al. A novel homozygous missense mutation in the insulin receptor gene results in an atypical presentation of Rabson-Mendenhall syndrome. Eur J Med Genet. 2016;59:16–9.
67. Gupta J, Daniel JM, Vasudevan V. Rabson-Mendenhall syndrome. J Indian Soc Pedodontics Preventive Dent. 2012;30:279.
68. Sinnarajah K, Dayasiri MBKC, Dissanayake NDW, Kudagammana ST, Jayaweera AHHM. Rabson Mendenhall syndrome caused by a novel missense mutation. Int J Pediatr Endocrinol. 2016;2016(1):21. https://doi.org/10.1186/s13633-016-0039-1.
69. Chong YH, Taylor BJ, Wheeler BJ. Renal manifestations of severe Rabson-Mendenhall syndrome: a case report. J Diabetes Metab Disord. 2013;12:7.
70. Fu Z, Gilbert ER, Liu D. Regulation of insulin synthesis and secretion and pancreatic Beta-cell dysfunction in diabetes. Curr Diabetes Rev. 2013;9:25–53.
71. Tokarz VL, MacDonald PE, Klip A. The cell biology of systemic insulin function. J Cell Biol. 2018;217:2273–89.
72. Henquin J-C. The dual control of insulin secretion by glucose involves triggering and amplifying pathways in β-cells. Diabetes Res Clin Pract. 2011;93(Suppl 1):S27–31.

73. Skelin Klemen M, Dolenšek J, Slak Rupnik M, Stožer A. The triggering pathway to insulin secretion: functional similarities and differences between the human and the mouse β cells and their translational relevance. Islets. 2017;9:109–39.
74. Rorsman P, Braun M. Regulation of insulin secretion in human pancreatic islets. Annu Rev Physiol. 2013;75:155–79.
75. Seino S, Shibasaki T, Minami K. Dynamics of insulin secretion and the clinical implications for obesity and diabetes. J Clin Invest. 2011;121:2118–25.
76. Singh B, Saxena A. Surrogate markers of insulin resistance: a review. World J Diabetes. 2010;1:36–47.
77. Satin LS, Butler PC, Ha J, Sherman AS. Pulsatile insulin secretion, impaired glucose tolerance and type 2 diabetes. Mol Asp Med. 2015;42:61–77.
78. Hou JC, Min L, Pessin JE. Insulin granule biogenesis, trafficking and exocytosis. Vitam Horm. 2009;80:473–506.
79. Tolliver S, Graham J, Kaffenberger BH. A review of cutaneous manifestations within glucagonoma syndrome: necrolytic migratory erythema. Int J Dermatol. 2018;57:642–5.
80. Huo J, Liu P, Chen X, Wu J, An J, Ren J. Delayed diagnosis of glucagonoma syndrome: a case report. Int J Dermatol. 2016;55:1272–4.
81. Corrias G, Horvat N, Monti S, Basturk O, Lin O, Saba L, et al. Malignant transformation of glucagonoma with SPECT/CT In-111 OctreoScan features: a case report. Medicine (Baltimore). 2017;96:e9252.
82. Tseng H-C, Liu C-T, Ho J-C, Lin S-H. Necrolytic migratory erythema and glucagonoma rising from pancreatic head. Pancreatology. 2013;13:455–7.
83. Albrechtsen NJW, Challis BG, Damjanov I, Jens JH. Do glucagonomas always produce glucagon? Bosn J Basic Med Sci. 2016;16:1–7.
84. Zhang K, Lehner LJ, Praeger D, Baumann G, Knebel F, Quinkler M, et al. Glucagonoma-induced acute heart failure. Endocrinol Diabetes Metab Case Rep. 2014;2014:140061. https://doi.org/10.1530/EDM-14-0061.
85. Demir OM, Paschou SA, Ellis HC, Fitzpatrick M, Kalogeropoulos AS, Davies A, et al. Reversal of dilated cardiomyopathy after glucagonoma excision. Hormones (Athens). 2015;14:172–3.
86. John AM, Schwartz RA. Glucagonoma syndrome: a review and update on treatment. J Eur Acad Dermatol Venereol. 2016;30:2016–22.
87. Ito T, Lee L, Jensen RT. Carcinoid-syndrome: recent advances, current status and controversies. Curr Opin Endocrinol Diabetes Obes. 2018;25:22.
88. Liu EH, Solorzano CC, Katznelson L, Vinik AI, Wong R, Randolph G. AACE/ACE disease state clinical review: diagnosis and management of midgut carcinoids. Endocr Pract. 2015;21:534–45.
89. Hannah-Shmouni F, Stratakis CA, Koch CA. Flushing in (neuro)endocrinology. Rev Endocr Metab Disord. 2016;17:373–80.
90. Matthes S, Bader M. Peripheral serotonin synthesis as a new drug target. Trends Pharmacol Sci. 2018;39:560–72.
91. Frazer A, Hensler JG. Chapter 13: serotonin receptors. In: Siegel GJ, Agranoff BW, Albers RW, Fisher SK, Uhler MD, editors. Basic neurochemistry: molecular, cellular, and medical aspects. Philadelphia: Lippincott-Raven; 1999. p. 263–92.
92. Kulke MH, Hörsch D, Caplin ME, et al. Telotristat ethyl, a tryptophan hydroxylase inhibitor for the treatment of carcinoid syndrome. JCO. 2016;35:14–23.
93. Biçer EN, Öztürk AB, Ozyigit LP, Erus S, Tanju S, Dilege Ş, et al. A case of uncontrolled severe asthma patient with coexisting carcinoid tumor presenting as pneumomediastinum. J Asthma. 2015;52:1095–8.
94. Bertino EM, Confer PD, Colonna JE, Ross P, Otterson GA. Pulmonary neuroendocrine/carcinoid tumors. Cancer. 2009;115:4434–41.
95. Hassan SA, Banchs J, Iliescu C, Dasari A, Lopez-Mattei J, Yusuf SW. Carcinoid heart disease. Heart. 2017;103:1488–95.

96. Savvidou S. Pellagra: a non-eradicated old disease. Clin Pract. 2014;4(1):637. https://doi.org/10.4081/cp.2014.637.
97. Crook MA. The importance of recognizing pellagra (niacin deficiency) as it still occurs. Nutrition. 2014;30:729–30.
98. Bell HK, Poston GJ, Vora J, Wilson NJE. Cutaneous manifestations of the malignant carcinoid syndrome. Br J Dermatol. 2005;152:71–5.
99. Kleyn CE, Bell H, Postin G, Wilson N. Cutaneous manifestations of the malignant carcinoid syndrome1. J Am Acad Dermatol. 2004;50:P113.
100. Nikou GC, Angelopoulos TP. Current concepts on gastric carcinoid tumors. Gastroenterol Res Pract. 2012;2012:287825. https://doi.org/10.1155/2012/287825.
101. Hou W, Schubert ML. Treatment of gastric carcinoids. Curr Treat Options Gastroenterol. 2007;10:123–33.
102. Dierdorf SF. Carcinoid tumor and carcinoid syndrome. Curr Opin Anaesthesiol. 2003;16:343–7.
103. Soga J. The term "carcinoid" is a misnomer: the evidence based on local invasion. J Exp Clin Cancer Res. 2009;28:15.
104. Oronsky B, Ma PC, Morgensztern D, Carter CA. Nothing but NET: a review of neuroendocrine tumors and carcinomas. Neoplasia. 2017;19:991–1002.
105. Abu-Zaid A, Azzam A, Abudan Z, Algouhi A, Almana H, Amin T. Sporadic pancreatic vasoactive intestinal peptide-producing tumor (VIPoma) in a 47-year-old male. Hematol Oncol Stem Cell Ther. 2014;7:109–15.
106. Hagen BM, Bayguinov O, Sanders KM. VIP and PACAP regulate localized Ca2+ transients via cAMP-dependent mechanism. Am J Phys Cell Phys. 2006;291:C375–85.
107. Tang B, Yong X, Xie R, Li Q-W, Yang S-M. Vasoactive intestinal peptide receptor-based imaging and treatment of tumors (Review). Int J Oncol. 2014;44:1023–31.
108. Fujiya A, Kato M, Shibata T, Sobajima H. VIPoma with multiple endocrine neoplasia type 1 identified as an atypical gene mutation. BMJ Case Rep. 2015;2015:bcr2015213016. https://doi.org/10.1136/bcr-2015-213016.
109. Berna MJ, Hoffmann KM, Serrano J, Gibril F, Jensen RT. Serum gastrin in Zollinger-Ellison syndrome: I. prospective study of fasting serum gastrin in 309 patients from the National Institutes of Health and comparison with 2229 cases from the literature. Medicine (Baltimore). 2006;85:295–330.
110. Remme CA, de Groot GH, Schrijver G. Diagnosis and treatment of VIPoma in a female patient. Eur J Gastroenterol Hepatol. 2006;18:93–9.
111. Apodaca-Torrez FR, Triviño M, Lobo EJ, Goldenberg A, Triviño T. Extra-pancreatic vipoma. Arq Bras Cir Dig. 2014;27:222–3.
112. Da Silva XG. The cells of the islets of Langerhans. J Clin Med. 2018;7(3):54. https://doi.org/10.3390/jcm7030054.
113. Brereton MF, Vergari E, Zhang Q, Clark A. Alpha-, Delta- and PP-cells. J Histochem Cytochem. 2015;63:575–91.
114. Kiriyama Y, Nochi H. Role and cytotoxicity of amylin and protection of pancreatic islet β-cells from amylin cytotoxicity. Cell. 2018;7(8):95. https://doi.org/10.3390/cells7080095.
115. Briant L, Salehi A, Vergari E, Zhang Q, Rorsman P. Glucagon secretion from pancreatic α-cells. Ups J Med Sci. 2016;121:113–9.
116. Iki K, Pour PM. Distribution of pancreatic endocrine cells including IAPP-expressing cells in non-diabetic and type 2 diabetic cases. J Histochem Cytochem. 2007;55:111–8.
117. Napolitano T, Silvano S, Vieira A, Balaji S, Garrido-Utrilla A, Friano ME, et al. Role of ghrelin in pancreatic development and function. Diabetes Obes Metab. 2018;20(Suppl 2):3–10.
118. Smith JP, Fonkoua LK, Moody TW. The role of gastrin and CCK receptors in pancreatic cancer and other malignancies. Int J Biol Sci. 2016;12:283–91.
119. Shin JJ, Gorden P, Libutti SK. Insulinoma: pathophysiology, localization and management. Future Oncol. 2010;6:229–37.
120. Zhang WD, Liu DR, Wang P, Zhao JG, Wang ZF, Chen L. Clinical treatment of gastrinoma: a case report and review of the literature. Oncol Lett. 2016;11:3433–7.

121. Ligiero Braga T, Santos-Oliveira R. PPoma review: epidemiology, aetiopathogenesis, prognosis and treatment. Diseases. 2018;6(1):8. https://doi.org/10.3390/diseases6010008.
122. Williamson J, Thorn C, Spalding D, Williamson R. Pancreatic and peripancreatic somatostatinomas. Ann R Coll Surg Engl. 2011;93:356–60.
123. Tsoukalas N, Chatzellis E, Rontogianni D, Alexandraki KI, Boutzios G, Angelousi A, et al. Pancreatic carcinoids (serotonin-producing pancreatic neuroendocrine neoplasms). Medicine. 2017;96(16):e6201. https://doi.org/10.1097/MD.0000000000006201.
124. La Rosa S, Franzi F, Albarello L, Schmitt A, Bernasconi B, Tibiletti MG, et al. Serotonin-producing enterochromaffin cell tumors of the pancreas: clinicopathologic study of 15 cases and comparison with intestinal enterochromaffin cell tumors. Pancreas. 2011;40:883–95.
125. Oberg K, Casanovas O, Castaño JP, et al. Molecular pathogenesis of neuroendocrine tumors: implications for current and future therapeutic approaches. Clin Cancer Res. 2013;19:2842–9.
126. Gaur P, Sceusi EL, Samuel S, et al. Identification of cancer stem cells in human gastrointestinal carcinoid and neuroendocrine tumors. Gastroenterology. 2011;141:1728–37.
127. Dai H, Hong X, Wang X, Lin C, Wu W, Zhao Y. Pancreatic neuroendocrine tumor cancer stem cells: potential novel therapeutic targets? Trans Cancer Res. 2016;5:860–70.

Parathyroid Gland and Musculoskeletal Signs

5

Learning Objectives

At the end of this chapter, you will be able to:

1. Recognize the effects of hypercalcemia and hypocalcemia on various organs
2. Understand the role of parathyroid hormone (PTH) in osteoclastogenesis
3. Understand the mechanisms underlying the classic Albright hereditary osteodystrophy phenotype of pseudohypoparathyroidism
4. Understand the pathophysiologic basis for the clinical features of Paget's disease of the bone
5. Understand the pathophysiology of vitamin D-resistant rickets and hypophosphatemic rickets

5.1 Hyperparathyroidism

5.1.1 Acute Abdomen

Clinical Features

Hyperparathyroidism can cause a myriad of nonspecific abdominal complaints and may sometimes present as an acute abdomen. Acute pancreatitis and complications of hypergastrinemia, e.g., peptic ulcer disease, may result in an acute surgical abdomen [1]. Acute pancreatitis has been associated with hyperparathyroidism since it was first described in the 1950s [1]. A study in 2006 reported a 28-fold increase in the risk of pancreatitis among patients with hyperparathyroidism when compared to controls in the general population [2].

© Springer Nature Switzerland AG 2020
A. Manni, A. Quarde, *Endocrine Pathophysiology*,
https://doi.org/10.1007/978-3-030-49872-6_5

Pathophysiology
The gastrointestinal manifestations of hyperparathyroidism are mediated by elevated serum calcium:

1. The association between hyperparathyroidism and hypergastrinemia could be due to multiple endocrine neoplasia syndrome type 1 or a direct causal relationship between serum calcium and gastrin levels [1].
2. Hypercalcemia due to underlying hyperparathyroidism may cause precipitation of calcium, which impairs drainage of the pancreatic ducts, leading to obstruction and inflammation of the pancreas. Also, hypercalcemia facilitates the conversion of inactive trypsinogen to active trypsin. Trypsin activation in the pancreas sets off an inflammatory cascade that culminates in acute pancreatitis [1].

5.1.2   Fragility Fractures

Clinical Features
Fragility fractures due to hyperparathyroidism in young subjects have been reported [3]. The loss of cortical bone mineral density is disproportionately higher than that of lamellar (cancellous) bone, making the distal third radius an ideal site to evaluate with bone densitometry in patients with this condition [4].

Pathophysiology
In normal physiology, PTH binds to osteoblasts and activates them through complex downstream processes. An activated osteoblast's surface-bound *receptor activator of nuclear factor κ-B ligand* (RANK-L) binds to *receptor activator of nuclear factor κ-B* (RANK) present on the surface of the osteoclast. This promotes osteoclast activation and subsequently leads to increased bone resorption. PTH also suppresses the synthesis of osteoprotegerin (OPG) – a soluble decoy receptor for RANK-L, which results in a higher number of RANK-Ls being available to bind osteoclast surface-bound RANK (see Fig. 5.1) [5–7].

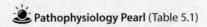 Pathophysiology Pearl (Table 5.1)

5.1.3   Band Keratopathy/Cataracts

Clinical Features
Band keratopathy is a clinical finding in various conditions, including hyperparathyroidism. It is a whitish-gray opacification involving the cornea with a predilection for the nasal or temporal regions of the cornea [12].

Pathophysiology
The underlying mechanism is yet to be elucidated. Hyperparathyroidism-induced hypercalcemia causes an increase in the solubility product of calcium and

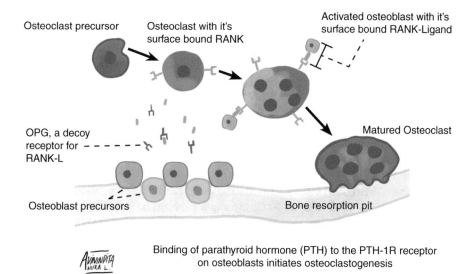

Osteoclast precursor

Osteoclast with it's
surface bound RANK

Activated osteoblast with it's
surface bound RANK-Ligand

OPG, a decoy
receptor for
RANK-L

Matured Osteoclast

Osteoblast precursors

Bone resorption pit

Binding of parathyroid hormone (PTH) to the PTH-1R receptor
on osteoblasts initiates osteoclastogenesis

Fig. 5.1 Schematic representation of PTH-mediated osteoblast-osteoclast interaction. PTH binds to the PTH-1R (parathyroid hormone 1 receptor) on osteoblasts; this is the first step in the eventual activation of osteoclasts. Osteoblast surface-bound RANK-L binds to RANK on osteoclasts leading to differentiation of an osteoclast precursor into a mature osteoclast. Mature osteoclasts present in bone resorption pits are responsible for the liberation of calcium sequestered in hydroxyapatite crystals. Osteoprotegerin is a soluble decoy receptor for RANK-L, which provides negative feedback inhibition of osteoclast activation [11]. (Redrawn and modified from Ikeda and Takeshita [11])

Table 5.1 Other clinical manifestations of hyperparathyroidism

Clinical finding	Mechanism
Pigeon chest (an exaggerated protrusion of the anterior chest)	Multiple vertebral fractures [8]
Shortened distal phalanges	PTH-mediated bone resorption [9]
Calciphylaxis (tender, necrotic, and dark eschar involving the skin)	Soft tissue calcification due to a high calcium-phosphate solubility product promotes ischemia and necrosis [10]

Adapted from Sharma [8] Lachungpa [9] and Erdel [10]

phosphate, which leads to precipitation of calcium salts. This reported mechanism is supported by the presence of calcium salt depositions in Bowman's membrane of the cornea [12, 13].

5.1.4   Hypertension

Clinical Features

Hypertension is widely accepted as being associated with primary hyperparathyroidism. There is a reported prevalence of 20–80%, most likely due to study significant heterogeneity [14]. A large retrospective study involving more than 4000 subjects reported higher all-cause mortality and cardiovascular specific deaths when patients with primary hyperparathyroidism were compared to matched controls [15].

Pathophysiology
1. Elevated levels of PTH activate the renin-angiotensin-aldosterone system (RAAS). PTH causes an increase in renin secretion through a complex homeostatic system involving serum calcium, 25 hydroxyvitamin D, and renal 1α hydroxylase enzyme [16].
2. Binding of PTH to the PTH-1R receptors on the zona glomerulosa cells stimulates the release of aldosterone. Aldosterone mediates fluid and sodium retention, which leads to an increase in blood pressure [17].
3. PTH binding to cardiac myocyte surface-bound PTH-1R promotes hypertrophy of the cardiac myocytes due to an upregulation in gene expression and protein synthesis [18].
4. Hyperparathyroidism causes vasodilatation of vascular smooth muscle. At high concentrations of circulating PTH, there is a paradoxical impairment of PTH's vasodilatory effects. This is believed to be due to the release of endothelin-1 and IL-6, which promotes increased collagen formation, endothelial dysfunction, and eventual impairment of vasodilatation [16].

 Pathophysiology Pearl

The Role of the Calcium-Sensing Receptor Activation in Mediating Serum Calcium

Calcium Sensing receptor (CaSR) in the parathyroid gland: CaSR present on the cellular membrane of the chief cells of the parathyroid gland senses the level of extracellular calcium and regulates calcium concentration by influencing PTH synthesis [19].

Increasing amounts of extracellular ionized calcium activate the CaSR, which sets off a cascade of intracellular reactions (phospholipase C- and adenylate cyclase-mediated processes), which increases cytosolic calcium concentration. Calcium response elements (CRE) present on the PreProPTH gene detect the high intracellular calcium and downregulates the transcription and translation of PTH. *The net effect of CaSR activation in the parathyroid gland is, therefore, a reduction in PTH synthesis* [20].

Calcium Sensing receptor (CaSR) in the kidney: The CaSR present on the basolateral surface of the thick ascending limb of Henle's loop (TALH) is activated in the setting of hypercalcemia. Through various intracellular processes, there is a downregulation of potassium channels and the sodium-potassium adenosine triphosphatase (Na-K-ATPase). The necessary luminal positive electrical gradient required for the absorption of divalent cations such as magnesium and calcium is therefore impaired. This results in hypercalciuria and a reduction in serum calcium. The net effect of CaSR activation in the TALH is, therefore, a reduction in serum calcium [21].

Familial hypocalciuric hypercalcemia is an autosomal dominant disorder characterized by a *loss of function mutation of the CaSR gene*. The CaSR is, therefore, unable to sense the levels of ionized calcium in the extracellular fluid. At the level of the parathyroid gland, this results in PTH synthesis even in the setting of hypercalcemia. In the TALH, there is increased calcium conservation, which leads to mild hypercalcemia. Most patients with this condition are asymptomatic but may occasionally develop acute pancreatitis or cholelithiasis. An important endocrinology dictum requires all patients undergoing evaluation for primary hyperparathyroidism to have an assessment of 24-hour urinary calcium excretion. This will prevent inadvertent parathyroid gland exploration in patients with hypocalciuria in the setting of PTH-mediated hypercalcemia [22].

Autosomal dominant hypocalcemia with hypercalciuria (ADHH) is characterized by a gain of function mutation of the CaSR. As was previously mentioned, CaSR activation in the chief cells of the parathyroid gland reduces PTH synthesis and, in the TALH, promotes hypercalciuria. The biochemical phenotype is, therefore, similar to that of idiopathic hypoparathyroidism, i.e., hypocalcemia and hyperphosphatemia, however, with a low but detectable PTH [23]. Patients with ADHH develop significant suppression of PTH after calcium supplementation and are generally at an increased risk for nephrocalcinosis (see Sect. 5.2.1) [24, 25] (Table 5.2).

 Questions You Might Be Asked on Clinical Rounds

What is the classic bone manifestation of primary hyperparathyroidism?

Osteitis fibrosa cystica (OFC) is a rare bone manifestation of severe primary hyperparathyroidism [26, 27] with a reported prevalence between 2% and 5% in developed countries [28]. This classic lesion of primary hyperparathyroidism can sometimes present with a pathologic fracture and may be misdiagnosed as a malignancy [27, 29]. OFC can be challenging to distinguish from malignancy, based on radiologic features alone [29].

Histologically it has been described as a focus of extensive bone remodeling, characterized by significant osteopenia, fibrosis, and hemorrhage. Hemosiderin deposition due to the breakdown of red blood cells gives it the

Table 5.2 The effect of calcium-sensing receptor mutations on PTH secretion and renal calcium conservation

	Pathophysiology	PTH	Serum calcium
FHH	Loss-of-function mutation of the CaSR	Increased PTH synthesis and secretion	Hypercalcemia due to increased renal calcium reabsorption [22]
ADHH	Gain-of-function mutation of the CaSR	Decreased PTH synthesis and secretion	Hypocalcemia due to reduced renal calcium reabsorption [23]

ADHH Autosomal dominant hypocalcemia with hypercalciuria, *FHH* Familial hypocalciuric hypercalcemia, *CaSR* Calcium sensing receptor, *PTH* Parathyroid hormone
Adapted from Papadopoulou [22] and Roszko [23]

classic brown discoloration, widely referred to as "brown tumors" [27]. Lesions of OFC tend to involve the jaw bone, long bones, ribs, and pelvis [30].

What are the skeletal effects of parathyroid hormone (PTH)?

PTH preferentially reduces cortical (compact) bone mineral density at a rate higher than that of cancellous (trabecular) bone. The distal radius has the highest content of cortical bone, making it an ideal site for estimating the effects of PTH on bone via bone densitometry [31] (Table 5.3).

What are the mechanisms underlying the various causes of hypercalcemia?

Idiopathic Causes of Hypercalcemia

Idiopathic hypercalcemia is characterized by elevated levels of 1,25 dihydroxy vitamin D (calcitriol), hypercalciuria with or without hypophosphatemia. Mutations in the CYP24A and SLC34A1 are associated with idiopathic hypercalcemia [40, 41] (Table 5.4).

Table 5.3 Mechanisms of the causes of hypercalcemia

Mechanism	Cause of hypercalcemia
Increased osteoclast-mediated bone resorption	Hyperparathyroidism [32]
	Hyperthyroidism [32]
	PTHrp-mediated hypercalcemia [33]
	Lithium (increased PTH set point)
	Prolonged period of immobilization [32]
	Hypervitaminosis A [34]
Increased gastrointestinal calcium absorption (calcitriol mediated)	Lymphomas [33]
	Tuberculomas [35]
	Sarcoidosis [36]
	Histoplasmosis [35]
	Berylliosis [35]
	Silicone-implant (foreign body granuloma) [37, 38]
	Williams syndrome (increased sensitivity to vitamin D metabolites) [39]
Increased renal conservation of calcium	Inactivating mutation of the CaSR (familial hypocalciuric hypercalcemia) [32]
	Thiazides [32]
	Hypervitaminosis D [32]

CaSR Calcium sensing receptor, *PTH* Parathyroid hormone, *PTHrp* Parathyroid hormone-related peptide
Adapted from Refs. [32–39]

Table 5.4 Inactivating gene mutations recently identified in patients with idiopathic hypercalcemia

Gene	Physiological role	Clinical features
SLC34A1 (autosomal recessive)	This gene encodes the renal sodium phosphate transporter, pivotal in renal phosphate conservation	Hypophosphatemia results in reduced Fibroblast growth factor 23 (FGF-23) production (a potent 1alpha hydroxylase inhibitor). Increased calcitriol promotes gut absorption of both calcium and phosphate [41]
CYP24A (autosomal recessive)	This gene encodes the 24-hydroxylase enzyme which inactivates calcitriol	Calcitriol-mediated increased intestinal calcium and phosphate absorption [40]

Adapted from Schlingmann [40] and Schlingmann [41]

5.2   Hypoparathyroidism

5.2.1   Trousseau's Sign and Chvostek Sign in the Setting of Hypocalcemia

Clinical Features

Trousseau's sign usually manifests as limb spasms, best elicited by placing the cuff of a sphygmomanometer over the upper arm and inflating it to at least 20 mmHg above the systolic blood pressure [42–44]. It is both sensitive and specific for clinically significant hypocalcemia [42]. A study reported the prevalence of Trousseau's sign as being up to 94% in patients with biochemically confirmed hypocalcemia, compared with 1% in patients with normal serum calcium [45].

Dr. Franz Chvostek first reported a case of latent tetany in 1870 [46]. Chvostek's sign is a unilateral twitching of the facial musculature due to the tapping of the superficial part of the facial nerve. Percussion of the facial nerve can either be done anterior to the external acoustic meatus or directly on the cheek [46].

In contrast to Trousseau's sign, Chvostek's sign has poor specificity and sensitivity for hypocalcemia [42]. A systematic review reported the sensitivity of Chvostek's sign as ranging from 0% to 100% with a specificity of 78.8–100% among patients with hypocalcemia [46].

Pathophysiology
1. Extracellular calcium is critical in maintaining the permeability of sodium channels on neuronal cells. Hypocalcemia increases the influx of sodium and promotes neuronal excitability due to the lowering of the action potential threshold. This state of neuromuscular excitability is further aggravated by mechanical percussion of the peripheral part of the facial nerve (Chvostek's sign) [45].
2. Mild hypoxemia due to ischemia within the soft tissues distal to the inflated sphygmomanometer cuff causes Trousseau's sign [45].

5.2.2   Seizures

Clinical Features

Hypocalcemia-induced seizures can be a presentation of hypoparathyroidism, although any perturbation in calcium homeostasis irrespective of the underlying cause can result in seizures [47].

Pathophysiology

Hypocalcemia increases neuronal excitability through various effects on multiple neuronal ion channels, including voltage-gated sodium channels, calcium-activated potassium channels, and GABA receptors. This ultimately increases excitatory postsynaptic currents, accounting for the seizures observed in patients with clinically significant hypocalcemia [47].

5.2.3 Hypotension

Clinical Features
A case of hypocalcemia-induced hypotension was reported in a letter published in the *Journal of the American Medical Association* (JAMA) in 1972. The patient had refractory hypotension in the setting of uremic pericardial effusion and symptomatic hypocalcemia. Interestingly, the correction of hypocalcemia led to prompt resolution of hypotension before the performance of pericardiocentesis [48]. There have been other reports of hypocalcemia-induced hypotension since then [49, 50].

Pathophysiology
1. Calcium plays a critical role in the electrical-contraction-coupling cycle of cardiac myocytes. Reduced contractility of cardiac myocytes is a possible explanation for a low cardiac output in patients with hypocalcemia [49, 51].
2. QT prolongation due to hypocalcemia also increases the risk of arrhythmia-induced hypotension [49].

5.2.4 Papilledema

Clinical Features
Papilledema, a rare fundoscopic finding in patients with severe hypocalcemia, is characterized by a blurring of the optic disk margin [52].

Pathophysiology
Hypocalcemia increases adenylate cyclase activity in the choroid plexus and promotes the secretion of cerebrospinal fluid (CSF). An increase in CSF pressure around the optic nerve head leads to impaired perfusion to the neuron and eventual neuronal cell death [53].

 Questions You Might Be Asked on Clinical Rounds

What is the pathophysiologic basis of ectopic basal ganglia calcifications (Fahr's syndrome) in chronic hypoparathyroidism?

Impaired activity of renal sodium-phosphate transporters results in the accumulation of inorganic phosphate in the extracellular fluid compartment. It is worthy to note that phosphate accumulation increases the calcium-phosphate product, a significant risk factor for ectopic calcification [54]. Ectopic calcifications may also present as cataracts and nephrolithiasis [55, 56].

How does hypocalcemia cause pustular psoriasis?

1. Calcium-sensing receptors present on keratinocytes play an essential role in the differentiation and proliferation of keratinocytes and other skin appendages [57].
2. Cell adhesion molecules called cadherins require calcium for their optimal function; hypocalcemia impairs the function of cadherins and predisposes patients to pustular psoriasis [58].

There are case reports of pustular psoriasis in patients with primary hypo-parathyroidism, with the lesions resolving in response to correction of hypo-calcemia [59, 60]. To further substantiate the role of calcium in the pathogenesis of pustular psoriasis, calcium channel blockers are a known precipitating cause of psoriasis. In such scenarios, prompt discontinuation of these agents resulted in the resolution of skin lesions [61].

5.3   Pseudohypoparathyroidism

5.3.1   Short Stature

Clinical Features
Short stature is a cardinal clinical finding in Albright hereditary osteodystrophy (AHO). The classic AHO phenotype is characterized by round facies, obesity, brachydactyly, and short stature [62].

Pathophysiology
Short stature in patients with pseudohypoparathyroidism (PHP) occurs due to rapid chondrocyte differentiation leading to premature closure of the growth plate and eventual stunting of growth [63].

Impaired activity of Gsα affects PTH-mediated signaling in chondrocytes. This is even more profound during puberty and accounts for the short stature observed in patients with pseudohypoparathyroidism [64].

☀ **Pathophysiology Pearl**
PTH binds to the PTH-1R receptor, which leads to dissociation of Gsα from the heterotrimeric G protein. Gsα subsequently activates adenylyl cyclase (AC). This is followed by AC-mediated conversion of ATP to cyclic AMP. The second messenger, cyclic AMP activates protein kinase A

(PKA), which subsequently phosphorylates various target proteins involved in transcription and translation of several downstream cyclic AMP-responsive genes. A loss-of-function mutation involving the gene encoding the alpha subunit of the Gs protein, i.e., GNAS gene, results in *pseudohypoparathyroidism* [64].

Resistance to PTH action in the proximal renal tubule leads to hypocalcemia and hyperphosphatemia, a biochemical profile akin to what is observed in patients with isolated hypoparathyroidism. Patients, however, have a paradoxical elevation in serum PTH, hence the name, pseudohypoparathyroidism [64].

5.3.2 Obesity

Clinical Features
Most adults with PHP1A have a body mass index (BMI) >25 kg/m^2 [64]. The reported prevalence of obesity is more than 66%, higher than the 32% prevalence rate reported for the general population [65].

Pathophysiology
1. Melanocortin signaling pathways that regulate satiety are dependent on Gsα activity. Gsα activity is defective in PHP, which leads to impaired satiety, ultimately leading to obesity [64].
2. There are β adrenergic receptors in adipose tissue, which presumably play a role in lipolysis. Downstream signaling of these receptors is dependent on Gsα activity; as such, decreased fat mobilization occurs in patients with PHP [66].
3. Growth hormone (GH) deficiency is a contributory factor as well since growth hormone-releasing hormone (GHRH) signaling is dependent on the stimulatory G-protein, Gsα [65].

5.3.3 Brachydactyly

Clinical Features
The characteristic skeletal feature of PHP happens to be shortening of the metacarpals and metatarsals. This skeletal change tends to involve the fourth and fifth metacarpals and metatarsals [64, 67].

Pathophysiology
Impaired activity of Gsα affects parathyroid hormone-related peptide (PTHrp)-mediated signaling critical in chondrocyte proliferation in the growth plate [64].

5.3.4   Dental Manifestations

Clinical Features
Multiple dental abnormalities including delayed or even failed eruption of the teeth, blunting of the roots, hypodontia, and ankylosis [64, 68]. Patients should be referred to dentists for optimal care of the teeth [68].

Pathophysiology
Downstream signaling for PTH-1R in the tooth is affected due to impaired Gsα activity. This highlights the vital role of PTH in mediating tooth maturation and mineralization [64].

> ☀ **Pathophysiology Pearl**
>
> Pseudopseudohypoparathyroidism (PPHP)
>
>   This is a unique clinical and biochemical subtype of inactivating PTH/PTHrp signaling disorders (iPPSDs). The new iPPSD nomenclature acknowledges the spectrum of clinicopathologic phenotypes in patients with pseudohypoparathyroidism [69].
>
>   The *Guanine nucleotide binding protein, alpha stimulating* (GNAS) gene is critical in the transcription of the stimulatory G protein (Gsα). Gsα in most tissues is expressed in a biallelic fashion, i.e., there are distinct paternal and maternal alleles. The clinical and biochemical features are, therefore, dependent on the parent of origin of the mutant allele [70].
>
>   The paternal Gsα gene in normal physiology is not expressed in the proximal renal tubule, pituitary gland, and gonadal tissue. It, therefore, plays no role in renal electrolyte (calcium and phosphorus) handling or activation of Gsα-coupled receptors such as luteinizing hormone (LH), parathyroid hormone (PTH), and thyroid-stimulating hormone (TSH). An affected child who inherits a mutated Gsα gene from a father will, therefore, present with PPHP (i.e., short stature with no apparent biochemical or hormonal perturbations) [70].
>
>   Maternal Gsα gene expression, on the other hand, ultimately determines the downstream effects of Gsα-coupled receptors, including LH, PTH, TSH, and GHRH. Also, unlike the paternal allele, the maternal allele is expressed in pituitary, renal, and gonadal tissues. A mutation in the maternal Gsα gene, therefore, results in the classic pseudohypoparathyroidism type 1A (PHP1A) phenotype (see Table 5.5) [71, 72].
>
>   Pseudohypoparathyroidism type 1B (PHP1B) occurs when there is an imprinting (methylation) defect in the maternal GNAS gene. It is worthy to note that, in contrast to PPHP and PHP1A, there is no mutation in the Gsα gene [73].

Table 5.5 Clinical and biochemical features of some forms of iPPSD

iPPSD	AHO	Other hormone resistance states	PTH resistance
PPHP	Present	Absent	Absent [74, 75]
PHP1A	Present	Present	Present [71, 72]
PHP1B	Absent	Infrequent	Present [73]
PHP1C	Present	Present	Present [62]

iPPSD inactivating *PTH/PTHrp* signaling disorders, *AHO* Albright's hereditary osteodystrophy
Other hormone resistance states LH and TSH resistance
PTH resistance low calcium, high phosphorus and a paradoxically high PTH
PHP1C Pseudohypoparathyroidism type 1C
Adapted from Refs. [62, 71–75]

 Questions You Might Be Asked on Clinical Rounds

What is the classic phenotype of AHO?

Dr. Fuller Albright first described Albright hereditary osteodystrophy (AHO) in 1942. The classic phenotype has the following features, *brachydactyly, short stature*, and *round facies*. The classification system for this group of inactivating PTH/PTHrp signaling disorders is based on the presence or absence of the classic AHO phenotype and Gsα activity in response to exogenous PTH administration [69].

What are the other endocrinopathies which might be associated with some forms of pseudohypoparathyroidism?

- Resistance to the effects of TSH at the level of the thyroid gland results in hypothyroidism.
- Gonadotropin resistance leading to delayed puberty, oligomenorrhea, and cryptorchidism.
- Growth hormone-releasing hormone (GHRH) resistance causes GH deficiency.
- Prolactin deficiency.

Interestingly, ACTH, CRH, and vasopressin action are not affected in iPPSDs, because both the maternal and paternal copies of the GNAS gene are expressed in these tissues, as such a mutation in one parental allele does not result in hormonal defects since the normal parental allele is present. This highlights the tissue-specific expression of both maternal and paternal copies of the gene [76].

5.4   Paget's Disease of Bone

5.4.1 Fractures and Bone Deformity

Clinical Features

Patients with Paget's disease of bone (PDB) have a significant clinical fracture prevalence ranging between 10% and 30%. They may either be incomplete fissure fractures involving part of the cortical bone or complete transverse fractures. Fractures typically affect weight-bearing bones, which have a pre-existing deformity [77]. Bowing deformities tend to involve weight-bearing long bones in the lower extremity [78]. Patients may also present with skull and facial deformities such as frontal bossing [79].

Pathophysiology
PDB starts as a focal area of increased osteoclastogenesis (bone resorption), which is then followed by rapid bone formation, a process that leads to improperly formed bone (woven bone). The affected bones are, therefore, unable to withstand mechanical stress and, as such, are prone to deformities and fractures [79]. The etiology of the insult, which sets off the inevitable skeletal changes, is incompletely understood [80, 81].

5.4.2 Congestive Heart Failure

Clinical Features
Heart failure can occur in patients with extensive pagetoid changes in the bone; it is, however, an uncommon presentation of PDB [80, 82].

Pathophysiology
PDB causes high output cardiac failure because increased vascularization of bones affected by pagetic changes results in a reflex increase in stroke volume. This leads to cardiac remodeling and eventual decompensation (Frank-Starling law of the heart) [83].

5.4.3 Sensorineural Hearing Loss

Clinical Features
Sensorineural hearing loss (SNHL) is a known neurologic complication of PDB involving the skull [84]. The classic Weber and Rinne tests, which involve the use of a tuning fork, can be used at the bedside to differentiate conductive from SNHL. The tests require the use of a 512 Hz (Hertz) tuning fork in assessing both bone and air conduction [85].

A recent systematic review evaluated the accuracy of the Weber and Rinne tests. It showed wide variability in the sensitivity and specificity of these tests since adherence to testing protocols were operator dependent [86]. We will refer readers to other clinical examination texts for the standard protocol of these tuning fork tests.

Interestingly it is reported that Ludwig van Beethoven suffered from PDB and that his SNHL may have influenced some of his musical compositions [87].

Pathophysiology
A double-blind prospective study in 2004 involving 64 subjects with Paget's disease of the skull evaluated the auditory thresholds and auditory brainstem responses. The extent of pagetoid involvement of the temporal bone, measured

by computed tomography, was compared to objectively measured levels of hearing loss. There was a statistically significant positive correlation between the extent of pagetoid involvement of the cochlear capsule and the degree of SNHL.

Pagetoid involvement of the cochlear capsule is the cause of SNHL and not the previously reported mechanism of auditory nerve compression [84].

 Questions You Might Be Asked on Clinical Rounds

What are the other cardiac manifestations of Paget's disease, apart from high output cardiac failure?

Aortic stenosis, atherosclerosis, and endocardial calcifications [77]

How are patients with PGD more likely to present?

Up to 70% of patients are asymptomatic due to a prolonged period of latency in PGD. In symptomatic patients, a dull and deep aching pain involving pagetic bones is a more likely complaint at presentation [88].

5.5   Hereditary Vitamin D-Resistant Rickets Type 2 (HVDRR-II)

5.5.1   Rickets

Clinical Features

Dr. Fuller Albright reported a case of vitamin D-resistant rickets in 1937. He postulated the underlying cause of rickets in his case report as being due to "an intrinsic resistance to the anti-rachitic action of vitamin D" [89]. The clinical features of rickets occur at a young age [90, 91] and classically manifests before fusion of the growth plates [92]. Rickets tends to affect the distal forearms, knees, and costochondral regions [93]. The typical features include swelling of the costochondral joints (rachitic rosary), widening of the wrist joint, and an exaggerated genu varum in children [94].

Pathophysiology

HVDRR-II is an autosomal recessive condition due to a mutation in the vitamin D receptor gene, which results in impaired activity of vitamin D due to end-organ resistance to the action of 1,25-dihydroxyvitamin D. Patients develop hypocalcemia with or without hypophosphatemia [95].

There is another form of vitamin D-dependent rickets, which is due to a mutation in the gene encoding the renal 1-alpha-hydroxylase enzyme [96].

Transformation of cartilage into bone involves a cycle of laying down of cartilage matrix, its resorption, and replacement by series of woven bone and then the eventual formation of mature lamellar bone. Mineralization of newly

Table 5.6 Pathophysiologic basis of other clinical features of rickets

Clinical feature	Underlying cause
Decreased linear growth	Impaired mineralization in the growth plate [94]
Tetany	Hypocalcemia [94]
Hypotonia	Hypocalcemia [94]
Recurrent respiratory infections	Hypotonia involving respiratory musculature results in an inability to clear airway secretions [94]

Adapted from Sahay and Sahay [94]

formed osteoid is defective due to lack of calcium and phosphorus [92], which results in the formation of defective bones unable to withstand mechanical stress. This leads to the typically exaggerated genu varum seen in rickets [93] (Table 5.6).

 Questions You Might Be Asked on Clinical Rounds

How can HVDRR-II be differentiated from vitamin D resistance due to 1α hydroxylase deficiency, biochemically?

Low serum calcium and phosphate with high parathyroid hormone levels occur in both conditions. 1,25 hydroxyvitamin D3 is, however, low in 1α hydroxylase deficiency but high in HVDRR [91].

What are the roles of the parathyroid gland, kidneys, and bone in calcium and phosphate homeostasis?

1. PTH promotes a net increase in serum calcium and decrease in serum phosphorus [97].
2. 1,25-Dihydroxy vitamin D3 promotes a net increase in both serum calcium and phosphorus [98].
3. FGF-23 promotes a net decrease in serum phosphate [99]. Refer to Fig. 5.2.

5.6   X-Linked Hypophosphatemic Rickets

5.6.1   Short Stature

Clinical Features

Patients with X-linked hypophosphatemic rickets (XLHR) have short stature, with the length of the lower limbs more significantly affected than that of the trunk. This results in an abnormal upper segment to lower segment ratio (lower segment = from the top of the symphysis pubis to the heel; upper segment = height minus lower segment) [101]. Early treatment with oral phosphate supplementation and calcitriol improves growth rates and other skeletal outcomes [102].

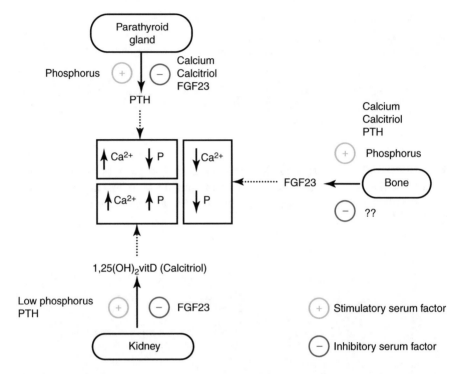

Fig. 5.2 The role of various hormones in calcium and phosphorus homeostasis. PTH facilitates the leaching of calcium from bone by mediating the activation of osteoclasts. In the kidney, PTH stimulates renal 1α hydroxylase activity (increased calcitriol production), which ultimately promotes reabsorption of calcium in the distal nephron and inhibits phosphate conservation in the proximal renal tubules [97]. 1,25-Dihydroxy vitamin D3 (active vitamin D) has various effects, including stimulation of osteoclast differentiation (bone), calcium conservation (distal renal tubule), phosphate conservation (proximal nephron), and calcium and phosphate reabsorption in the small intestine [98]. FGF-23 inhibits both phosphate conservation by the proximal renal tubule and 1α hydroxylase activity in the proximal renal tubule [99]. Hypophosphatemia and intravenous iron infusions have been reported as factors that inhibit the gene encoding FGF-23 [100]. Solid arrow from an organ (parathyroid gland, bone, and kidney) represents the active secretion of a hormone. Dotted arrow represents the effects of the designated hormone on serum calcium and phosphate levels. (Based on Goltzman et al. [97])

Pathophysiology

1. Growth plate activity is highest around the knees and determines the final skeletal height. Impaired endochondral bone formation due to significant hypophosphatemia accounts for a disproportionate shortening of the lower limbs compared to the upper limbs [103].
2. Mechanical loading of the lower extremities leads to the characteristic bowing of the legs and subsequent shortening of the patient's final height [103].

5.6.2   Dental Abscess

Clinical Features
Unprovoked dental abscesses occur in the absence of trauma or dental caries. Active dental surveillance to optimize oral hygiene is recommended, and there are no active therapies to prevent this complication [104].

Pathophysiology
Phosphate forms an essential component of hydroxyapatite crystals (mineralized bone). Evidence suggests that patients with XLHR have poor mineralization of the dentine layer of the tooth situated below the enamel. Eventual expansion of the pulp cavity leads to a breach in this protective dentine layer and predisposes patients to dental infections [105].

 Questions You Might Be Asked on Clinical Rounds

What is the role of fibroblast growth factor 23 (FGF-23) in calcium and phosphate homeostasis?

1. FGF-23 is a phosphaturic hormone secreted by osteocytes [105], which increases phosphate excretion at the level of the proximal tubule by inhibiting the expression of sodium-phosphate transporters needed in phosphate conservation [101].

   Also, it decreases 1α hydroxylation activity and potentiates 24α hydroxylation of vitamin D, leading to low levels of serum calcitriol [106, 107]. In theory, the physiologic effect of FGF-23 is a reduction in both renal and gastrointestinal phosphate absorption [108].

What is the underlying cause of X-linked hypophosphatemia (XLH)?
A mutation in the PHEX (phosphate-regulating gene with homologies to endopeptidase on the X chromosome) gene results in impaired expression of a peptidase involved in the inactivation of FGF-23. This promotes increased circulating levels of FGF-23, which causes hypophosphatemia and reduced bone mineralization [106].

There is a new FDA-approved monoclonal antibody for the treatment of XLH called burosumab. Burosumab binds circulating intact FGF23 and, thereby, blocks its biologic effects in target tissues. It improves renal tubular phosphate conservation and serum phosphorus levels and promotes linear growth [108].

An important differential diagnosis of XLH is *Tumor-induced osteomalacia* (TIO). TIO is caused by increased production of FGF-23 by mesenchymal tumors. FGF-23 causes reduced insertion of sodium phosphate channels in the renal tubules, which results in increased urinary loss of phosphorus. Besides, there is decreased production of calcitriol due to FGF-23-mediated inactivation of 1α hydroxylase activity (see Fig. 5.3). Additionally, affected patients develop poor bone mineralization due to significant hypophosphatemia [109].

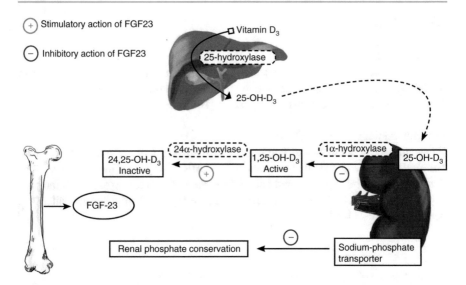

Fig. 5.3 The role of FGF-23 in positive and negative feedback pathways involved in vitamin D homeostasis. Vitamin D3 undergoes an initial hydroxylation step in the liver and is then transferred to the kidneys for 1 alpha hydroxylation (dashed arrow) [97]. The conversion of 25 hydroxyvitamin D3 to its active form, i.e., 1,25-dihydroxy vitamin D3, is inhibited by FGF-23. Also, FGF-23 facilitates the inactivation of active vitamin D into its inactive form, i.e., 24,25 dihydroxy vitamin D3, by potentiating the action of the 24-hydroxylase enzyme. The net effect is a reduction in the production of active vitamin D in the presence of FGF-23 [106, 107]. Furthermore, FGF-23 promotes renal phosphate loss [101]. (Based on Goltzman et al. [97])

References

1. Abboud B, Daher R, Boujaoude J. Digestive manifestations of parathyroid disorders. World J Gastroenterol. 2011;17:4063–6.
2. Jacob JJ, John M, Thomas N, Chacko A, Cherian R, Selvan B, Nair A, Seshadri MS. Does hyperparathyroidism cause pancreatitis? A south Indian experience and a review of published work. ANZ J Surg. 2006;76:740–4.
3. Ozaki A, Tanimoto T, Yamagishi E, et al. Finger fractures as an early manifestation of primary hyperparathyroidism among young patients: a case report of a 30-year-old male with recurrent osteoporotic fractures. Medicine (Baltimore). 2016;95:e3683.
4. Bilezikian JP. Primary hyperparathyroidism. J Clin Endocrinol Metabol. 2018;103:3993–4004.
5. Zhang S, Wang X, Li G, Chong Y, Zhang J, Guo X, Li B, Bi Z. Osteoclast regulation of osteoblasts via RANK-RANKL reverse signal transduction in vitro. Mol Med Rep. 2017;16:3994–4000.
6. Jilka RL, O'Brien CA, Bartell SM, Weinstein RS, Manolagas SC. Continuous elevation of PTH increases the number of osteoblasts via both osteoclast-dependent and -independent mechanisms. J Bone Miner Res. 2010;25:2427–37.
7. Park JH, Lee NK, Lee SY. Current understanding of RANK signaling in osteoclast differentiation and maturation. Mol Cells. 2017;40:706–13.
8. Sharma S, Kumar S. Bilateral genu valgum: an unusual presentation of juvenile primary hyperparathyroidism. Oxf Med Case Reports. 2016;2016:141–3.

9. Lachungpa T, Sarawagi R, Chakkalakkoombil SV, Jayamohan AE. Imaging features of primary hyperparathyroidism. BMJ Case Rep. 2014;2014:bcr2013203521. https://doi.org/10.1136/bcr-2013-203521.
10. Erdel BL, Juneja R, Evans-Molina C. A case of calciphylaxis in a patient with hypoparathyroidism and normal renal function. Endocr Pract. 2014;20:e102–5.
11. Ikeda K, Takeshita S. The role of osteoclast differentiation and function in skeletal homeostasis. J Biochem. 2016;159:1–8.
12. Kobayashi W, Yokokura S, Hariya T, Nakazawa T. Two percent ethylenediaminetetraacetic acid chelation treatment for band-shaped keratopathy, without blunt scratching after removal of the corneal epithelium. Clin Ophthalmol. 2015;9:217–23.
13. Weng S-F, Jan R-L, Chang C, Wang J-J, Su S-B, Huang C-C, Tseng S-H, Chang Y-S. Risk of band keratopathy in patients with end-stage renal disease. Sci Rep. 2016;6:28675.
14. Carrelli AL, Silverberg SJ. Primary hyperparathyroidism and hypertension. In: Koch CA, Chrousos GP, editors. Endocrine hypertension: underlying mechanisms and therapy. Totowa: Humana Press; 2013. p. 181–94.
15. Brown SJ, Ruppe MD, Tabatabai LS. The parathyroid gland and heart disease. Methodist Debakey Cardiovasc J. 2017;13:49–54.
16. Yao L, Folsom AR, Pankow JS, Selvin E, Michos ED, Alonso A, Tang W, Lutsey PL. Parathyroid hormone and the risk of incident hypertension: the Atherosclerosis Risk in Communities study. J Hypertens. 2016;34:196–203.
17. Brown J, de Boer IH, Robinson-Cohen C, Siscovick DS, Kestenbaum B, Allison M, Vaidya A. Aldosterone, parathyroid hormone, and the use of renin-angiotensin-aldosterone system inhibitors: the multi-ethnic study of atherosclerosis. J Clin Endocrinol Metab. 2015;100:490–9.
18. Schlüter KD, Piper HM. Cardiovascular actions of parathyroid hormone and parathyroid hormone-related peptide. Cardiovasc Res. 1998;37:34–41.
19. Chen RA, Goodman WG. Role of the calcium-sensing receptor in parathyroid gland physiology. Am J Physiol Renal Physiol. 2004;286:F1005–11.
20. Conigrave AD. The calcium-sensing receptor and the parathyroid: past, present. Future Front Physiol. 2016;7:563. https://doi.org/10.3389/fphys.2016.00563.
21. Riccardi D, Brown EM. Physiology and pathophysiology of the calcium-sensing receptor in the kidney. Am J Physiol Renal Physiol. 2010;298:F485–99.
22. Papadopoulou A, Gole E, Melachroinou K, Meristoudis C, Siahanidou T, Papadimitriou A. Identification and functional characterization of a calcium-sensing receptor mutation in an infant with familial Hypocalciuric Hypercalcemia. J Clin Res Pediatr Endocrinol. 2016;8:341–6.
23. Roszko KL, Bi RD, Mannstadt M. Autosomal dominant hypocalcemia (Hypoparathyroidism) types 1 and 2. Front Physiol. 2016;7:458. https://doi.org/10.3389/fphys.2016.00458.
24. Kim MY, Tan AHK, Ki C-S, et al. Autosomal dominant hypocalcemia caused by an activating mutation of the calcium-sensing receptor gene: the first case report in Korea. J Korean Med Sci. 2010;25:317–20.
25. Yamamoto M, Akatsu T, Nagase T, Ogata E. Comparison of hypocalcemic hypercalciuria between patients with idiopathic hypoparathyroidism and those with gain-of-function mutations in the calcium-sensing receptor: is it possible to differentiate the two disorders? J Clin Endocrinol Metab. 2000;85:4583–91.
26. Silverberg SJ, Bilezikian JP. Evaluation and management of primary hyperparathyroidism. J Clin Endocrinol Metab. 1996;81:2036–40.
27. Misiorowski W, Czajka-Oraniec I, Kochman M, Zgliczyński W, Bilezikian JP. Osteitis fibrosa cystica-a forgotten radiological feature of primary hyperparathyroidism. Endocrine. 2017;58:380–5.
28. Maina AM, Kraus H. Successful treatment of osteitis fibrosa cystica from primary hyperparathyroidism. Case Rep Orthop. 2012;2012:3. https://doi.org/10.1155/2012/145760.

29. Jervis L, James M, Howe W, Richards S. Osteolytic lesions: osteitis fibrosa cystica in the setting of severe primary hyperparathyroidism. BMJ Case Rep. 2017;2017:bcr-2017. https://doi.org/10.1136/bcr-2017-220603.
30. Mellouli N, Belkacem Chebil R, Darej M, Hasni Y, Oualha L, Douki N. Mandibular osteitis fibrosa cystica as first sign of vitamin D deficiency. Case Rep Dent. 2018;2018:5. https://doi.org/10.1155/2018/6814803.
31. Bilezikian JP, Brandi ML, Eastell R, Silverberg SJ, Udelsman R, Marcocci C, Potts JT. Guidelines for the management of asymptomatic primary hyperparathyroidism: summary statement from the Fourth International Workshop. J Clin Endocrinol Metab. 2014;99:3561–9.
32. Carroll R, Matfin G. Endocrine and metabolic emergencies: hypercalcaemia. Ther Adv Endocrinol Metab. 2010;1:225–34.
33. Mirrakhimov AE. Hypercalcemia of malignancy: an update on pathogenesis and management. N Am J Med Sci. 2015;7:483–93.
34. Vyas AK, White NH. Case of hypercalcemia secondary to hypervitaminosis a in a 6-year-old boy with autism. Case Rep Endocrinol. 2011;2011:424712. https://doi.org/10.1155/2011/424712.
35. Sharma OP. Hypercalcemia in granulomatous disorders: a clinical review. Curr Opin Pulm Med. 2000;6:442–7.
36. Burke RR, Rybicki BA, Rao DS. Calcium and vitamin D in sarcoidosis: how to assess and manage. Semin Respir Crit Care Med. 2010;31:474–84.
37. Yedla N, Perez E, Lagari V, Ayala A. Silicone granulomatous inflammation resulting in hypercalcemia: a review of the literature. AACE Clin Case Rep. 2018;5:e119–23.
38. Negri AL, Rosa Diez G, Del Valle E, Piulats E, Greloni G, Quevedo A, Varela F, Diehl M, Bevione P. Hypercalcemia secondary to granulomatous disease caused by the injection of methacrylate: a case series. Clin Cases Miner Bone Metab. 2014;11:44–8.
39. Sindhar S, Lugo M, Levin MD, et al. Hypercalcemia in patients with Williams-Beuren syndrome. J Pediatr. 2016;178:254–60.e4.
40. Schlingmann KP, Kaufmann M, Weber S, et al. Mutations in CYP24A1 and idiopathic infantile hypercalcemia. N Engl J Med. 2011;365:410–21.
41. Schlingmann KP, Ruminska J, Kaufmann M, et al. Autosomal-recessive mutations in SLC34A1 encoding sodium-phosphate cotransporter 2A cause idiopathic infantile Hypercalcemia. J Am Soc Nephrol. 2016;27:604–14.
42. Jesus JE, Landry A. Images in clinical medicine. Chvostek's and Trousseau's signs. N Engl J Med. 2012;367:e15.
43. Marcucci G, Cianferotti L, Brandi ML. Clinical presentation and management of hypoparathyroidism. Best Pract Res Clin Endocrinol Metab. 2018;32(6):927–39. https://doi.org/10.1016/j.beem.2018.09.007.
44. Chhabra P, Rana SS, Sharma V, Sharma R, Bhasin DK. Hypocalcemic tetany: a simple bedside marker of poor outcome in acute pancreatitis. Ann Gastroenterol. 2016;29:214–20.
45. Cooper MS, Gittoes NJL. Diagnosis and management of hypocalcaemia. BMJ. 2008;336:1298–302.
46. Hujoel IA. The association between serum calcium levels and Chvostek sign. Neurol Clin Pract. 2016;6:321–8.
47. Han P, Trinidad BJ, Shi J. Hypocalcemia-induced seizure. ASN Neuro. 2015;7(2) https://doi.org/10.1177/1759091415578050.
48. Chaimovitz C, Abinader E, Benderly A, Better OS. Hypocalcemic hypotension. JAMA. 1972;222:86–7.
49. Thurlow JS, Yuan CM. Dialysate-induced hypocalcemia presenting as acute intradialytic hypotension: a case report, safety review, and recommendations. Hemodial Int. 2016;20:E8–E11.
50. Ghent S, Judson MA, Rosansky SJ. Refractory hypotension associated with hypocalcemia and renal disease. Am J Kidney Dis. 1994;23:430–2.

51. Wong CK, Lau CP, Cheng CH, Leung WH, Freedman B. Hypocalcemic myocardial dysfunction: short- and long-term improvement with calcium replacement. Am Heart J. 1990;120:381–6.
52. Gradisnik P. Hypoparathyroidism should always be checked in papilledema. J Neurosci Rural Pract. 2017;8:329.
53. Goyal JL, Kang J, Gupta R, Anand A, Arora R, Jain P. Bilateral papilledema in hypocalcemia. Sci J. 2012;23:127–30.
54. Mitchell DM, Regan S, Cooley MR, Lauter KB, Vrla MC, Becker CB, Burnett-Bowie S-AM, Mannstadt M. Long-term follow-up of patients with hypoparathyroidism. J Clin Endocrinol Metab. 2012;97:4507–14.
55. Shoback D. Hypoparathyroidism. N Engl J Med. 2008;359:391–403.
56. Mendes EM, Meireles-Brandão L, Meira C, Morais N, Ribeiro C, Guerra D. Primary hypoparathyroidism presenting as basal ganglia calcification secondary to extreme hypocalcemia. Clin Pract. 2018;8(1):1007. https://doi.org/10.4081/cp.2018.1007.
57. Popp T, Steinritz D, Breit A, Deppe J, Egea V, Schmidt A, Gudermann T, Weber C, Ries C. Wnt5a/β-catenin signaling drives calcium-induced differentiation of human primary keratinocytes. J Invest Dermatol. 2014;134:2183–91.
58. Guerreiro de Moura CAG, de Assis LH, Góes P, Rosa F, Nunes V, Gusmão ÍM, Cruz CMS. A case of acute generalized pustular psoriasis of von Zumbusch triggered by hypocalcemia. Case Rep Dermatol. 2015;7:345–51.
59. Knuever J, Tantcheva-Poor I. Generalized pustular psoriasis: a possible association with severe hypocalcaemia due to primary hypoparathyroidism. J Dermatol. 2017;44:1416–7.
60. Stewart AF, Battaglini-Sabetta J, Millstone L. Hypocalcemia-induced pustular psoriasis of von Zumbusch. New experience with an old syndrome. Ann Intern Med. 1984;100:677–80.
61. Kitamura K, Kanasashi M, Suga C, Saito S, Yoshida S, Ikezawa Z. Cutaneous reactions induced by calcium channel blocker: high frequency of psoriasiform eruptions. J Dermatol. 1993;20:279–86.
62. Mantovani G, Bastepe M, Monk D, et al. Diagnosis and management of pseudohypoparathyroidism and related disorders: first international Consensus Statement. Nat Rev Endocrinol. 2018;14:476–500.
63. Hanna P, Grybek V, de Nanclares GP, et al. Genetic and epigenetic defects at the GNAS locus Lead to distinct patterns of skeletal growth but similar early-onset obesity. J Bone Miner Res. 2018;33:1480–8.
64. Linglart A, Levine MA, Jüppner H. Pseudohypoparathyroidism. Endocrinol Metab Clin N Am. 2018;47:865–88.
65. Long DN, McGuire S, Levine MA, Weinstein LS, Germain-Lee EL. Body mass index differences in pseudohypoparathyroidism type 1a versus pseudopseudohypoparathyroidism may implicate paternal imprinting of Gαs in the development of human obesity. J Clin Endocrinol Metab. 2007;92:1073–9.
66. Carel JC, Le Stunff C, Condamine L, Mallet E, Chaussain JL, Adnot P, Garabédian M, Bougnères P. Resistance to the Lipolytic action of epinephrine: a new feature of protein Gs deficiency. J Clin Endocrinol Metab. 1999;84:4127–31.
67. Linglart A, Fryssira H, Hiort O, et al. PRKAR1A and PDE4D mutations cause acrodysostosis but two distinct syndromes with or without GPCR-signaling hormone resistance. J Clin Endocrinol Metab. 2012;97:E2328–38.
68. Reis MTA, Matias DT, de Faria MEJ, Martin RM. Failure of tooth eruption and brachydactyly in pseudohypoparathyroidism are not related to plasma parathyroid hormone-related protein levels. Bone. 2016;85:138–41.
69. Turan S. Current nomenclature of pseudohypoparathyroidism: inactivating parathyroid hormone/parathyroid hormone-related protein signaling disorder. J Clin Res Pediatr Endocrinol. 2017;9:58–68.
70. Turan S, Bastepe M. GNAS spectrum of disorders. Curr Osteoporos Rep. 2015;13:146–58.

71. Thiele S, Mantovani G, Barlier A, et al. From pseudohypoparathyroidism to inactivating PTH/PTHrP signalling disorder (iPPSD), a novel classification proposed by the EuroPHP network. Eur J Endocrinol. 2016;175:P1–P17.
72. Mantovani G, Elli FM. Inactivating PTH/PTHrP signaling disorders. Parathyroid Disord. 2019;51:147–59.
73. Dixit A, Chandler KE, Lever M, Poole RL, Bullman H, Mughal MZ, Steggall M, Suri M. Pseudohypoparathyroidism type 1b due to paternal uniparental disomy of chromosome 20q. J Clin Endocrinol Metab. 2013;98:E103–8.
74. Elli FM, deSanctis L, Ceoloni B, Barbieri AM, Bordogna P, Beck-Peccoz P, Spada A, Mantovani G. Pseudohypoparathyroidism type Ia and pseudo-pseudohypoparathyroidism: the growing spectrum of GNAS inactivating mutations. Hum Mutat. 2013;34:411–6.
75. Simpson C, Grove E, Houston BA. Pseudopseudohypoparathyroidism. Lancet. 2015;385:1123.
76. Mantovani G. Pseudohypoparathyroidism: diagnosis and treatment. J Clin Endocrinol Metab. 2011;96:3020–30.
77. Paul Tuck S, Layfield R, Walker J, Mekkayil B, Francis R. Adult Paget's disease of bone: a review. Rheumatology (Oxford). 2017;56:2050–9.
78. Kang H, Park Y-C, Yang KH. Paget's disease: skeletal manifestations and effect of bisphosphonates. J Bone Metab. 2017;24:97–103.
79. Shaker JL. Paget's disease of bone: a review of epidemiology, pathophysiology and management. Ther Adv Musculoskelet Dis. 2009;1:107–25.
80. Whyte MP. Paget's disease of bone. N Engl J Med. 2006;355:593–600.
81. Falchetti A, Masi L, Brandi ML. Paget's disease of bone: there's more than the affected skeletal–a clinical review and suggestions for the clinical practice. Curr Opin Rheumatol. 2010;22:410–23.
82. Singer FR, Bone HG, Hosking DJ, Lyles KW, Murad MH, Reid IR, Siris ES. Paget's disease of bone: an endocrine society clinical practice guideline. J Clin Endocrinol Metab. 2014;99:4408–22.
83. Palleschi L, Nunziata E. Severe congestive heart failure in elderly patient with Paget's disease. Geriatric Care. 2017;3(1) https://doi.org/10.4081/gc.2017.6727.
84. Monsell EM. The mechanism of hearing loss in Paget's disease of bone. Laryngoscope. 2004;114:598–606.
85. Rasgon B, Schloegel LJ. Early and accurate diagnosis of sudden sensorineural hearing loss. Perm J. 2009;13:61–3.
86. Kelly EA, Li B, Adams ME. Diagnostic accuracy of tuning fork tests for hearing loss: a systematic review. Otolaryngol Head Neck Surg. 2018;159:220–30.
87. Oiseth SJ. Beethoven's autopsy revisited: a pathologist sounds a final note. J Med Biogr. 2017;25:139–47.
88. Alonso N, Calero-Paniagua I, del Pino-Montes J. Clinical and genetic advances in Paget's disease of bone: a review. Clinic Rev Bone Miner Metab. 2017;15:37–48.
89. Albright F, Butler AM, Bloomberg E. Rickets resistant to vitamin D therapy. Am J Dis Child. 1937;54:529–47.
90. Choudhury S, Jebasingh KF, Ranabir S, Singh TP. Familial vitamin D resistant rickets: end-organ resistance to 1,25-dihydroxyvitamin D. Indian J Endocrinol Metab. 2013;17:S224–7.
91. Malloy PJ, Feldman D. Genetic disorders and defects in vitamin d action. Endocrinol Metab Clin North Am. 2010;39:333–46.
92. Pettifor JM. Rickets and vitamin D deficiency in children and adolescents. Endocrinol Metab Clin N Am. 2005;34:537–53, vii.
93. Wharton B, Bishop N. Rickets. Lancet. 2003;362:1389–400.
94. Sahay M, Sahay R. Rickets–vitamin D deficiency and dependency. Indian J Endocrinol Metab. 2012;16:164–76.
95. Malloy PJ, Zhou Y, Wang J, Hiort O, Feldman D. Hereditary vitamin D-resistant rickets (HVDRR) owing to a heterozygous mutation in the vitamin D receptor. J Bone Miner Res. 2011;26:2710–8.

96. Zalewski A, Ma NS, Legeza B, Renthal N, Flück CE, Pandey AV. Vitamin D-dependent rickets type 1 caused by mutations in CYP27B1 affecting protein interactions with adrenodoxin. J Clin Endocrinol Metab. 2016;101:3409–18.

97. Goltzman D, Mannstadt M, Marcocci C. Physiology of the calcium-parathyroid hormone-vitamin D axis. Front Horm Res. 2018;50:1–13.

98. Christakos S, Dhawan P, Verstuyf A, Verlinden L, Carmeliet G. Vitamin D: metabolism, molecular mechanism of action, and pleiotropic effects. Physiol Rev. 2016;96:365–408.

99. Erben RG. Physiological actions of fibroblast growth factor-23. Front Endocrinol. 2018;9:267. https://doi.org/10.3389/fendo.2018.00267.

100. Fukumoto S. Targeting fibroblast growth factor 23 signaling with antibodies and inhibitors, is there a rationale? Front Endocrinol (Lausanne). 2018;9:48.

101. Santos F, Fuente R, Mejia N, Mantecon L, Gil-Peña H, Ordoñez FA. Hypophosphatemia and growth. Pediatr Nephrol. 2013;28:595–603.

102. Meyerhoff N, Haffner D, Staude H, et al. Effects of growth hormone treatment on adult height in severely short children with X-linked hypophosphatemic rickets. Pediatr Nephrol. 2018;33:447–56.

103. Zivičnjak M, Schnabel D, Billing H, et al. Age-related stature and linear body segments in children with X-linked hypophosphatemic rickets. Pediatr Nephrol. 2011;26:223–31.

104. Carpenter TO, Imel EA, Holm IA, Jan de Beur SM, Insogna KL. A clinician's guide to X-linked hypophosphatemia. J Bone Miner Res. 2011;26:1381–8.

105. Carpenter TO. The expanding family of hypophosphatemic syndromes. J Bone Miner Metab. 2012;30:1–9.

106. Prié D, Friedlander G. Genetic disorders of renal phosphate transport. N Engl J Med. 2010;362:2399–409.

107. Reilly RF. Tumor-induced osteomalacia. J Onconephrol. 2018;2(2–3):92–101.

108. Lyseng-Williamson KA. Burosumab in X-linked hypophosphatemia: a profile of its use in the USA. Drugs Ther Perspect. 2018;34:497–506.

109. Chong WH, Molinolo AA, Chen CC, Collins MT. Tumor-induced osteomalacia. Endocr Relat Cancer. 2011;18:R53–77.

Reproductive Organ Signs

6

Learning Objectives
At the end of this chapter, you will be able to:

1. Discover the pathophysiologic mechanisms underlying the classic Turner's syndrome phenotype
2. Recognize the signs of hyperandrogenism seen in polycystic ovarian syndrome (PCOS)
3. Understand the hypothalamic-pituitary-gonadal axis
4. Identify the clinical features of the female menopausal state
5. Identify hormone resistance states involving estrogens and androgens and their unique clinical manifestations

6.1 Turner's Syndrome

6.1.1 Short Stature

Clinical Features
Short stature is a measured height of less than −2.5 standard deviations below the mean for the general population. It is a common clinical finding in patients with Turner's syndrome (TS). In a recent study involving 176 girls with Turner's syndrome, the midparental height was sensitive and served as a valuable tool in assessing short stature in children [1]. Growth failure during childhood results in a predictable short stature in adult life. The average height of women with untreated TS is about 4 feet, 8 inches [2].

Pathophysiology

Mutations in the *SHOX gene (short-stature homeobox-containing gene)*, which is present on the short arm of the X chromosome, is responsible for the short stature observed in patients with TS. There are two inherited copies of the SHOX gene in normal women; one is on the active and the other on the inactive copy of the X chromosome. This allows the gene to escape the effects of lyonization. Furthermore, genetic males also possess the SHOX gene on their Y chromosomes. The ultimate determinant of height is, therefore, dose-dependent with regard to the SHOX gene [3]. SHOX gene is expressed in mesenchymal tissue and is responsible for chondroblast development in long bones of the upper and lower extremities. A single remaining copy of the SHOX gene (haploinsufficiency), as occurs in TS, is unable to facilitate the growth of long bones. This accounts for the eventual short stature of patients with Turner's syndrome [4, 5].

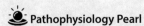 **Pathophysiology Pearl**

1. Mosaics 45,XO with (46,XX) may present with normal puberty and spontaneous menarche due to less severe ovarian defects, but almost universally have a short stature due to SHOX gene insufficiency [6].
2. TS patients with SHOX gene "overdosage," may present with tall stature. The reasons for this include the following:

- There is sustained growth of long bones due to an excess of this important osteogenic factor, i.e., SHOX gene.
- Gonadal dysgenesis leads to hypoestrogenemia and delayed fusion of the epiphyseal plate, leading to continuous growth. It is worthy to note that estrogen is critical in promoting fusion of the growth plate, a step required for cessation of vertical growth.

Interestingly the effect of the SHOX gene in determining final height is much more significant than hypoestrogenemia. Therefore, TS patients with overdosage of the SHOX gene will continue to grow even after initiating estrogen replacement therapy [3].

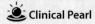 **Clinical Pearl**

What are the musculoskeletal monitoring recommendations for patients with TS?

1. Examine annually for scoliosis or even six-monthly, if a patient is on growth hormone supplementation therapy [7].
2. Monitor bone mineral density every 5 years when patients are on estrogen replacement therapy [7].

6.1.2 Webbed Neck and Lymphedema

Clinical Features
Patients with TS have a characteristic webbed neck (pterygium colli). Swelling of the hands and feet is also noted in infancy and facilitates early diagnosis of this condition [8].

Pathophysiology
Hypoplasia or aplasia of the lymphatic system causes impaired lymphatic drainage. Cervical lymphedema manifests clinically as a webbed neck [8].

 Clinical Pearl
What are the screening recommendations regarding hypothyroidism and celiac disease in patients with TS?

1. Annual screening for hypothyroidism [7].
2. Celiac screening is recommended every 2 years [7].

6.1.3 Hypertension

Clinical Features
Arterial hypertension has a reported prevalence of 13–58% in adult patients with TS. This confers a higher than fourfold increase in the risk of hypertension-related mortality in this patient population [9].

Pathophysiology
1. TS patients have significant metabolic comorbidities, including obesity, endothelial dysfunction, and hyperlipidemia, factors that increase the risk of hypertension [9, 10].
2. Activation of the renin-angiotensin-aldosterone axis has been proposed as a possible cause of hypertension in patients with TS [9].
3. Coarctation of the aorta and abnormal aortic arch morphology are contributing factors [9, 10].
4. Congenital renal abnormalities, e.g., horseshoe kidneys, predispose TS patients to recurrent infections, renal fibrosis, and secondary hypertension [9].

 Clinical Pearl
What are the cardiovascular screening recommendations for patients with TS?

1. Annual assessment of blood pressure, glycated hemoglobin, and fasting lipid profile [7].
2. In patients older than 16 years of age, annual transthoracic echocardiography, or cardiac MRI, is recommended due to the risk of aortic root dilatation [7].

6.1.4   Melanocytic Nevi

Clinical Features
Melanocytic nevi have a reported prevalence of 25–100%. These pigmented nevi tend to increase in size and number over time, with an increased risk of malignant transformation when they reach a size greater than 5–10 mm [11].

Pathophysiology
The pathophysiologic basis of melanocytic nevi (MN) is multifactorial. Genetics, sunlight exposure, and sex hormones are possible reasons for MN formation. The mechanisms involved in the development of MN, however, remain unclear at this time [11, 12].

6.1.5   Sexual Infantilism

Clinical Features
Girls with TS at the time of puberty are usually amenorrheic with no secondary sexual characteristics; however, those with mosaicism may develop primordial follicles in their ovaries, leading to estrogen-mediated breast development and hypomenorrhea [6].

Pathophysiology
The degree of gonadal dysgenesis is due to chromosomal pairing failure involving a region of the long arm of the X chromosome (Xq13-q26) during meiotic prophase. The greater the pairing anomaly, the more severe the extent of eventual gonadal dysgenesis and hypoestrogenemia [13].

 Questions You Might Be Asked on Clinical Rounds

Why are patients with Turner's syndrome at risk for diabetes mellitus?

Haploinsufficiency of the X chromosome affects genes encoding critical proteins involved in glucose sensing (glucokinase) or target tissue effects of insulin (hepatic nuclear factors). This results in impaired insulin secretion in response to hyperglycemia.

These defects contribute to progressive weight gain (due to hyperinsulinemia), which promotes peripheral insulin resistance. Patients progress through a stage of glucose intolerance before developing overt type 2 diabetes mellitus [14].

Which endocrinopathies are common in patients with Turner's syndrome?

Ovarian failure, autoimmune thyroid disease, type 1 or 2 diabetes, dyslipidemia, and osteopenia [15]

6.2 Polycystic Ovarian Syndrome

6.2.1 Hirsutism

Clinical Features

Hirsutism is defined as the presence of terminal, pigmented hair in a male pattern distribution. It is a common dermatologic manifestation of polycystic ovary syndrome (PCOS) with a reported prevalence of 50–70% [16].

The original assessment of hirsutism using the Ferriman-Gallwey score assigned a grade ranging from 0 to 4, depending on the presence and extent of terminal hair distribution involving 11 anatomic sites [17].

The forearm and lower leg have been excluded in the modified score since terminal hair growth in these areas is inconsistently associated with hyperandrogenemia. The modified Ferriman-Gallwey score objectively assesses nine anatomic regions for evidence of terminal hair growth [18]. A modified Ferriman-Gallwey score of ≥8 is consistent with clinically significant hirsutism [19, 20].

Pathophysiology

Circulating androgens are responsible for hirsutism, although the degree of hirsutism is not necessarily determined by the severity of hyperandrogenemia. This has been attributed to interindividual differences in the response of hair follicles to androgens [16] (see Sect. 1.1.5).

Hirsutism, like acne, and male pattern alopecia are dependent on the local abundance of 5α-reductase (which reduces testosterone to active dihydrotestosterone) in the pilosebaceous unit [21].

The local concentration of 5α-reductase in the skin varies by ethnicity. For example, hirsutism tends to be more common in women of Mediterranean background and less frequent and milder in women of East Asian or Native American background [22–24].

Endocrine Conditions Associated with Virilization

- Adrenal tumors.
- Cushing's syndrome.
- Classic and nonclassic congenital adrenal hyperplasia.
- Hyperandrogenism, insulin resistance, and acanthosis nigricans (*HAIR-AN syndrome*).
- Ovarian hyperthecosis.
- Ovarian tumors.
- The features of *virilization* include acne, male pattern baldness, deep male voice, and clitoral enlargement [25].

6.2.2 Acanthosis Nigricans

Clinical Features
Acanthosis nigricans (AN) is a classic dermatologic manifestation of PCOS and other endocrinopathies associated with insulin resistance. It is a velvety, dark, and plaque-like skin lesion which has a predilection for flexural areas such as the neck and axillary regions. 50% of patients with the classic obese PCOS phenotype have AN [26].

Pathophysiology
Hyperinsulinemia stimulates keratinocytes and fibroblasts directly, leading to their proliferation [26]. Additional mechanisms accounting for hyperinsulinemia-induced hirsutism have been described earlier (see also Sect. 4.1.1).

6.2.3 Acne

Clinical Features
Acne is a common skin manifestation of PCOS, with a highly variable prevalence, based on ethnicity. Asian Indians have the highest prevalence, with the lowest being among Pacific Islanders [27].

Pathophysiology
1. Hyperinsulinemia in the setting of PCOS potentiates the excretion of sebum through the effects of insulin acting on IGF-1 receptors present on sweat glands [16]. Accumulation of sebum establishes a milieu conducive for the proliferation of *Propionibacterium acnes* and eventual formation of comedones [28].
2. Dihydrotestosterone (an androgen) binds to its receptors on sweat glands and influences their output of sebum, as well [29]. Interestingly, the severity of acne is not dependent on the degree of hyperandrogenemia and may be due to the variable sensitivity of pilosebaceous units to circulating androgens [30].

6.2.4 Obesity

Clinical Features
The prevalence of obesity in patients with PCOS is between 40 and 80%. In contrast to women outside the USA, PCOS patients in the USA have relatively higher body mass indexes (BMIs) [31].

Pathophysiology
Circulating levels of androgen influence the distribution of body fat. Men have higher levels of testosterone and, as such, have a higher concentration of fat in the central abdomen compared to the hips or lower body.

Women with PCOS have high levels of testosterone, which changes the typical gynoid fat distribution into an android one. This is the reason for increased central or visceral adiposity [31].

More recent evidence refutes this hypothesis in women with PCOS. Although obese and nonobese women with PCOS had high levels of androgens compared to matched controls without PCOS, there was no difference in visceral adiposity between these two groups of PCOS subjects in this study [32]. The mechanisms remain incompletely understood at this time.

☀️ Pathophysiology Pearl

Pathogenesis of PCOS (Fig. 6.1)

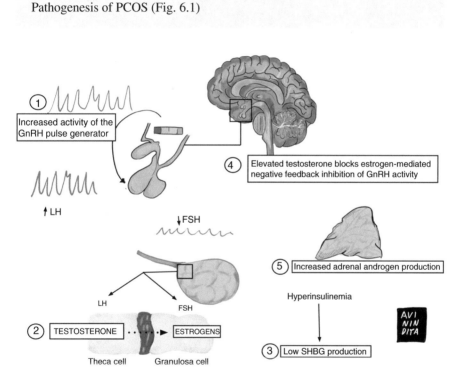

Fig. 6.1   Schematic representation of the pathophysiologic basis of PCOS. Step 1: Increased activity of the GnRH pulse generator stimulates central gonadotrophs and results in an increase in luteinizing hormone (LH) with a concomitant decrease in follicle-stimulating hormone (FSH) [33, 34]. Step 2: LH stimulates theca cells of the ovaries to produce testosterone. Low FSH, on the other hand, results in less stimulation of the granulosa cell-mediated conversion of theca cell-derived testosterone into estrogens [35]. Step 3: Reduced levels of circulating sex hormone-binding globulin (SHBG) [36] worsen the degree of hyperandrogenemia, as well. Both hyperandrogenemia and hyperinsulinemia impair hepatic SHBG synthesis [37], and since SHBG binds more avidly to estrogens than it does androgens, low levels of circulating SHBG increase the free androgen to free estrogen ratio. Step 4: Hyperandrogenemia impairs negative feedback effects of estrogen on the pituitary gonadotrophs, which results in unimpaired LH release and maintenance of a vicious cycle of hyperandrogenemia [38]. Step 5: Adrenal-derived androgens play a contributory role, although the mechanisms are incompletely understood [39]. (Redrawn and modified from Chaudhari et al. [34])

Questions You Might Be Asked on Clinical Rounds

What are the reasons for insulin resistance in patients with PCOS?

1. Post-insulin to insulin receptor binding defects contributes to insulin resistance in patients with PCOS [40].
2. Reduction in glucose transporter 4 (GLUT-4) receptors in adipose tissue leads to reduced glucose uptake [40].
3. Persistent hyperglycemia promotes rebound and *persistent hyperinsulinemia.* A prolonged period of hyperinsulinemia leads to progressive beta-cell dysfunction and death [40].
4. Androgens may play a modest role in insulin resistance, although elevated serum androgens alone cannot explain insulin resistance in PCOS [40].
5. Comorbid dyslipidemia contributes to lipotoxicity-induced insulin resistance [41].
6. There is also an increase, partially obesity-related, in inflammatory adipokines such as tumor necrosis factor alpha (TNF-α), which induces insulin resistance. Furthermore, there is a concomitant decrease in the insulin-sensitizing adipokine, adiponectin [42, 43].

What conditions should be ruled out as part of the evaluation of PCOS?
Hypothyroidism, prolactinoma, nonclassic congenital adrenal hyperplasia, Cushing's syndrome, androgen-secreting tumor, and acromegaly. Also, it is prudent to rule out pregnancy, primary ovarian insufficiency, or functional hypothalamic amenorrhea in select patients based on the clinical presentation [44]. It should go without saying that pregnancy must always be excluded in any woman of reproductive age with amenorrhea.

6.3   Male Hypogonadism

6.3.1   Decreased Testicular Volume

Clinical Features
Testicular volume (TV) is a valuable surrogate marker of testosterone production and spermiogenesis function [45]. Decreased testicular volume is associated with male hypogonadism and is more likely in primary hypogonadism compared to secondary hypogonadism [46].

The Prader orchidometer is an objective means of assessing testicular volume clinically. A cross-sectional study of over 400 subjects showed a strong, statistically significant positive correlation between clinical assessment of testicular volume using an orchidometer and ultrasound estimates [47].

Considerable tact and excellent reassurance skills are essential when using an orchidometer in order to prevent the patient from feeling inadequate.

A recent study evaluated the association between serum testosterone levels and adult testicular volumes in patients with either primary or secondary hypogonadism. A testicular volume of >30 cc, estimated by an orchidometer combined with BMI measurements, had a high predictive value in assessing if testosterone levels were optimal. TV combined with BMI had a sensitivity and specificity of 85.3% and 86.5%, respectively [45].

Pathophysiology
More than 90% of the testicular volume is accounted for by the quantity of sperm-producing seminiferous tubules. Testicular size is, therefore, predictive of spermiogenesis potential. Leydig cells do not contribute substantially to the final testicular volume; therefore, perturbations in seminiferous tubule function can result in a significant reduction in testicular size independent of Leydig cell function [48].

FSH and intratesticular testosterone promote the development of Sertoli cells (SCs), which are present on the epithelial cells of the seminiferous tubules. LH, on the other hand, stimulates the Leydig cells of the testes, which are responsible for the synthesis of testosterone [49].

In the setting of male hypogonadism, low levels of testosterone result in less trophic stimulation of the Sertoli cells present in the testis, leading to their eventual atrophy. This explains the low TV observed in patients with male hypogonadism [50].

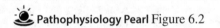 **Pathophysiology Pearl** Figure 6.2

 Clinical Pearl
What is the normal adult testicular size?
4 to 5.5 cm in length × 2.5 cm in width × 3 cm in the anteroposterior dimension.
The volume is reported as being greater than 20 ml in whites and African Americans [55] (Fig. 6.3).

6.3.2   Gynecomastia

Clinical Features
Gynecomastia is the presence of palpable glandular breast tissue in men [56] and should be differentiated from pseudogynecomastia, which is an enlargement of the breasts due to an accumulation of fat [57]. Gynecomastia is a reported finding in male hypogonadism [46].

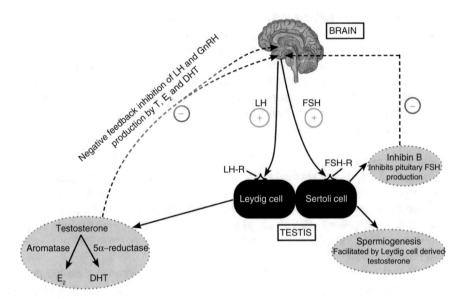

Fig. 6.2 Schematic diagram of the hypothalamic-pituitary-testicular axis. Gonadotropin-releasing hormone (GnRH) produced from the hypothalamus directly stimulates pituitary gonadotropes to release FSH and LH. LH binds to the G-protein-coupled LH receptor (LH-R) on the Leydig cell and stimulates the formation of testosterone [51]. Testosterone (T) is then converted to estradiol and dihydrotestosterone (DHT) by peripheral aromatase and the 5α-reductase enzymes, respectively (solid lines) [52]. Negative feedback inhibition of both gonadotropes and hypothalamic GnRH neurons is mediated by testosterone and estradiol (E2) (broken lines) [53]. FSH binds to the G-protein-coupled FSH receptor (FSH-R) on the Sertoli cell of the testis, a process that promotes the formation of sperms (spermatogenesis), androgen-binding proteins (ABPs), and inhibin B (solid lines). Spermatogenesis in the Sertoli cell is indeed under trophic stimulation by Leydig cell-derived testosterone [50]. Inhibin B suppresses FSH release from pituitary gonadotropes through a negative feedback loop (broken lines) [54]. (Based on Shalet [51])

Fig. 6.3 The Prader orchidometer. The objective assessment of testicular volume requires the use of an orchidometer – sequential beads labeled with an estimated testicular volume. Palpation and inspection of the testes facilitate an approximation of testicular volume, by comparing it to the beads on the orchidometer [45]. (Based on Ruiz-Olvera et al. [45])

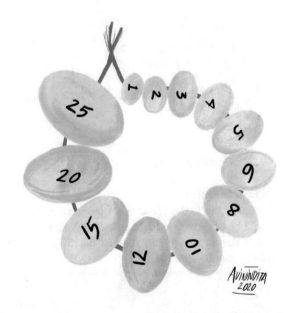

Pathophysiology
There are multiple receptors in the male breast for sex hormones and prolactin. In theory, estrogens stimulate the formation of the glandular breast tissue, while androgens lead to their regression. A tilt in the balance, in favor of estrogen, causes gynecomastia [56].

6.3.3 Loss of Height or Fragility Fractures

Clinical Features
Male hypogonadism contributes to a low bone mineral density, which can present as a fragility fracture [46]. The prevalence of secondary osteoporosis or osteopenia in patients with male hypogonadism remains unclear at this time [58].

Pathophysiology
1. Estrogen plays a vital role in maintaining bone mass in both adult males and females by inhibiting osteoclast activity (bone resorption). In males, testosterone is converted to estrogen by the aromatase enzyme present in adipose tissue. Testosterone, therefore, exerts indirect beneficial effects on bone mineral density [59].
2. Reduced muscle bulk and strength predispose hypogonadal men to falls, which increases their fracture risk [60].

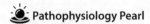 Pathophysiology Pearl
Aromatase Deficiency and Estrogen Resistance
   There is a single case report to date of a male with estrogen resistance and a clinical phenotype similar to that of men with congenital aromatase deficiency.

Clinical Features
- Tall stature with eunuchoid proportions due to persistent growth into adulthood
- Delayed bone age
- Low bone mineral density

Pathophysiology
Estrogen promotes skeletal maturation, epiphyseal fusion, the arrest of linear growth (in the peripubertal period), and maintenance of bone mineral density in adulthood. Typically, subjects with estrogen resistance or aromatase deficiency do not gain these beneficial effects of estrogen on skeletal metabolism [61].

6.3.4   Change in Body Composition

Clinical Features
Patients with male hypogonadism are predisposed to low muscle mass and strength in mainly the lower extremities [62].

For the most part, hypogonadism is associated with an increase in abdominal fat, which explains the increased waist-to-hip ratio seen in subjects with hypogonadism [63].

Pathophysiology
Low testosterone causes a reduction in muscle protein synthesis, which contributes to reduced muscle mass [63].

Testosterone inhibits lipoprotein lipase activity in adipose tissue. In male hypogonadism, the low levels of testosterone are unable to inhibit lipoprotein lipase activity; this results in increased lipid storage [63]. (see Sect. 1.4.1).

 Questions You Might Be Asked on Clinical Rounds

What are the clinical features of Klinefelter's syndrome (KS)?
Klinefelter's syndrome is characterized by features of *hypogonadism* (low libido, infertility, sparse androgenic hair growth), *gynecomastia, tall stature, and small testes* [64] (Table 6.1).

What is the genetic basis of Klinefelter's syndrome, and how is it different from 46,XX testicular disorder of sex development?
KS, a cause of *hypergonadotropic hypogonadism*, occurs in the setting of an XXY karyotype (extra X chromosome). Lyonization or inactivation of the X chromosome [67] may be somewhat incomplete, resulting in the expression of some residual active genes from the incompletely inactivated extra X chromosome [68].

80–90% of patients with KS have the *47,XXY genotype*. Other karyotypes which occur in KS include *48,XXXY, 48,XXYY*, or mosaics (*coexistence of 47,XXY and normal 46,XY*). These less common karyotypes account for up to 20% of patients [65].

In contrast to KS patients, who tend to be tall, males with 46,XX testicular disorder of sex development present with short stature due to paternal inheritance of an abnormal X chromosome [69].

During meiosis in the male parent, part of the Y chromosome material becomes affixed to the X chromosome. The sex-determining region of the Y chromosome (SRY) gene, which affects sex differentiation, is transferred to the defective X chromosome. The male infant has a normal male external genitalia, due to the presence of the SRY region; however, the azoospermia factor (AZF) region, which is critical in mediating spermiogenesis, becomes defective during meiosis in the affected parent. The affected male offspring develops oligospermia as a consequence of inheriting a defective azoospermic factor [70].

Table 6.1 The mechanisms underlying other clinical features of KS

Clinical feature(s)	Mechanism(s)
Loss of facial, chest, and pubic hair	Androgen deficiency [65]
Eunuchoid body habitus (arm span > height; waist-to-floor > waist-to-crown)	Testosterone deficiency and delayed epiphyseal closure due to hypoestrogenemia [65]
Absent frontal hair recession	Androgen deficiency [65, 66]

Adapted from Bonomi [65] and Urysiak-Czubatka [66]

6.4 Menopause

6.4.1 Vaginal Dryness

Clinical Features
Vaginal dryness is a known manifestation of menopause and has a reported prevalence ranging from 8% to 43% [71, 72]. Patients have other vulvovaginal signs, including shortening of the vagina and uterovaginal prolapse [73].

Pathophysiology
1. Hypoestrogenemia results in thinning of the vaginal mucosa due to low levels of local estrogen in the superficial cells of the vagina [74, 75]. The normal thick and moist vaginal mucosa is converted into a thin epithelium as a consequence of hypoestrogenemia [76].
2. Reduction in mucosal blood flow impairs vulvovaginal secretions [76].

6.4.2 Fragility Fractures

Clinical Features
The most important risk factor for low bone mineral density (BMD) in older women is menopause. The estimates of low postmenopausal BMD are as high as 40% depending on age and ethnicity. Fragility fractures are lower in postmenopausal African American women, compared to their age-matched Caucasian controls. African American postmenopausal women tend to have higher cortical and trabecular BMD than Caucasians, and this may be the reason for their low fracture rates [77].

Pathophysiology
1. Estrogen deficiency accelerates the rate of osteoclastogenesis (contributes to a significant decline in bone mineral density) [78].
2. Estrogen plays a critical role in preventing osteoblast apoptosis [78].
3. FSH spikes contribute to accelerated bone loss by stimulating osteoclastogenesis, especially in late premenopause and early menopause. Interestingly, women with central (low FSH) rather than primary hypogonadism (high FSH) lose less bone mineral density [79, 80].

6.4.3 Change in Body Composition

Clinical Features
Menopause is associated with increased central (visceral) adipose tissue deposition [81–83]. Postmenopausal women have a higher waist-to-hip ratio when compared to premenopausal controls. Indeed, in a study involving 358 women, central adiposity was more likely to be present in postmenopausal women, even after controlling for confounders such as the body mass index [84].

Pathophysiology
1. There is a predictable reduction in resting energy expenditure (REE), which mirrors estrogen levels in postmenopausal women [82]. A decline in REE results in reduced oxidation of fat [82] and leads to the accumulation of visceral and subcutaneous adipose tissue [81].
2. Estrogen causes accumulation of fat in the femoro-gluteal region, while androgens influence abdominal fat distribution. In postmenopausal women, a low estrogen state causes a reduction in hepatic production of sex hormone-binding globulin (SHBG). Low SHBG increases the levels of unbound active androgens. A shift in the balance toward androgens accounts for the central accumulation of fat observed in the postmenopausal period [85].

 Questions You Might Be Asked on Clinical Rounds

What are hot flashes in the menopausal age group?

Hot flashes happen to be the most prevalent symptom experienced by women during the climacteric [86]. Hot flashes present as intermittent periods of localized heat sensation, flushing (erythema), and excessive sweating involving the face and chest. The majority of patients experience amelioration of symptoms within 2 years [87].

Approximately 10% of patients might experience persistent bothersome hot flashes 10 years after their last menstrual period [88]. Discontinuation of hormone replacement therapy (HRT) may result in the resumption of symptomatic hot flashes at any time after menopause. Hot flashes are consistently associated with GnRH and FSH spikes and are generally not an issue in women with central hypogonadism (normal or low FSH) [89].

What are the cardioprotective effects of estrogen?

1. 17β-Estradiol increases the rate of ApoA-I synthesis (high-density lipoprotein) while decreasing the rate of ApoB-100 synthesis (triglyceride-laden lipoproteins) [90](see Fig. 7.2).
2. Estrogen increases the expression of LDL receptors on the surface of cells, which improves LDL clearance from peripheral tissues [91].
3. Estrogen directly increases the activity of lipoprotein lipase (lipid storage) and reduces the activity of hormone-sensitive lipase (lipid release) in adipose tissue (see Sect. 1.4.1) [90].

6.5   Estrogen Resistance

6.5.1   Tall Stature

Clinical Features
Tall stature was described in an index case of estrogen resistance in a male patient [92]. A recent case series including two females and one male, however, reported tall stature as an inconsistent finding in estrogen resistance [93]. Estrogen resistance is a rare condition with very few published case reports, making the exact estimation of prevalence uncertain [94].

Pathophysiology
Estrogen promotes both early pubertal growth spurt and subsequent closure of the epiphysis in late puberty [92]. The rate of attainment of final skeletal height is dependent on growth plate senescence (fusion), which is mediated by estrogen acting on its cognate receptors on chondrocytes [95, 96]. Estrogen plays this critical role in both males and females [61].

Mutation of the estrogen receptor leads to insensitivity to estrogen, resulting in impaired growth plate senescence [93]. Delayed growth plate fusion contributes to tall stature in these patients [97].

6.5.2   Acanthosis Nigricans

Clinical Features
Acanthosis nigricans (AN) was reported in an index case estrogen resistance in a male patient. The lesions were distributed in the bilateral axillae [92].

Pathophysiology
The reason for AN in the setting of insulin resistance and glucose intolerance was unexpected, although the authors proposed a possible reason for this clinical finding [92].

An increase in circulating estrogens improves glycemic control by facilitating insulin secretion and improving its target tissue effects. Due to acquired defects in estrogen receptors, estrogen is unable to play this physiological role, leading to insulin resistance [92].

 Questions You Might Be Asked on Clinical Rounds
What are the clinical features of females with estrogen resistance? [98]

- Low bone mineral density
- Impaired breast development
- Delayed puberty
- Lack of epiphyseal closure leading to tall stature

We have discussed the clinical features of classic estrogen resistance in the context of the estrogen receptor-α gene (ESR1); there has been a recently reported mutation of the estrogen receptor-β (ESR2). What are the clinical features of this recently described ESR2 mutation in a female patient?

- Streak ovaries
- Absent puberty
- Absent breast development
- Infantile uterus
- Osteoporosis with closed epiphysis

In contrast to patients with classic ESR1 mutations, patients with estrogen resistance due to ESR2 mutations have streak ovaries because the ESR2 receptor signaling pathway is critical for the differentiation and growth of the ovaries [98, 99].

6.6   Complete Androgen Insensitivity

6.6.1   Abnormalities of the External and Internal Genitalia

Clinical Features
Patients with complete androgen insensitivity have a short vagina with an absent cervix on pelvic examination [100]. Due to the normal-appearing female external genitalia, the diagnosis is often delayed [101].

Pathophysiology (Fig. 6.4)

6.6.2   Normal Breast Tissue Development

Clinical Features
Patients with CAIS usually have normal female breast tissue development [104]. Aberrant breast tissue anywhere along the mammary line has been reported as well [105]. There is spontaneous breast development around puberty; as such, patients can grow up with a female gender identity [106].

The standard practice is to bring up CAIS subjects as females, although there is a recent case of gender dysphoria in a 17-year-old patient with CAIS. The patient underwent female-to-male gender reassignment surgery and subsequently received gender-affirming hormone therapy [107].

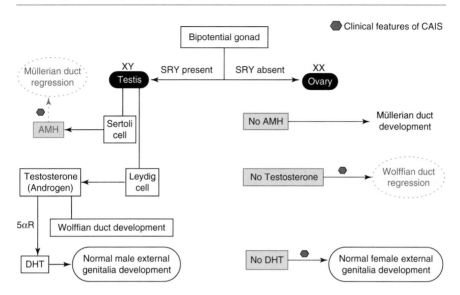

Fig. 6.4 Schematic diagram of normal differentiation of the bipotential gonad and the implications of complete androgen insensitivity. Complete androgen insensitivity syndrome (CAIS) occurs as a result of a mutation of the gene responsible for the translation of the androgen receptor (AR) [102, 103]. In utero, the bipotential gonad differentiates into either male or female gonad with ultimate phenotypic features being under the influence of the transcription factor, SRY (sex-determining region of the Y chromosome), androgens, and anti-Mullerian hormone (AMH) [104]. In a genetic male (XY), the SRY transcription factor present on the short arm of the Y chromosome plays a pivotal role in the differentiation of the bipotential gonad into a testis. AMH secreted by the Sertoli cells of the testis causes regression of the Mullerian ducts, which are responsible for the formation of the upper female genital structures (upper one-third of the vagina, uterus, and fallopian tubes) [104]. Androgens from the testes bind to androgen receptors and mediate the development of the Wolffian duct into male internal genital structures (seminal vesicles, epididymis, and vas deferens). Due to the mutation of the AR, the Wolffian ducts regress as well, leading to the formation of the lower female genitalia (lower two-third of the vagina, labia, and clitoris) [104]. (*SRY* sex-determining region of the Y chromosome, *5aR* 5 alpha-reductase). (Redrawn and modified from Hughes et al. [104])

Pathophysiology

Aromatization of androgens into estrogen promotes breast tissue development in patients with CAIS [103].

 Clinical Pearl

What are the other clinical features of CAIS? [106]

   Primary amenorrhea, inguinal hernias, and sparse or absent pubic and axillary hair

Questions You Might Be Asked on Clinical Rounds

Why should patients with CAIS and undescended testes undergo orchiectomy?

The risk of malignancy of an abdominally located testes increases with age, with an anticipated risk of malignancy of 3.6% at 25 years and an even higher risk of 33% by 50 years of age [108].

Why do patients with CAIS have incomplete or minimal axillary and pubic hair?

Vellus (nonpigmented or nonsexual) hair may be found in the pubic and axillary areas because it is not androgen-dependent. Darker terminal hair, which happens to be androgen-dependent, is, however, sparse or absent in CAIS. The inability of androgens to act at the hair root due to mutation of the androgen receptor accounts for these findings [109].

References

1. Ouarezki Y, Cizmecioglu FM, Mansour C, Jones JH, Gault EJ, Mason A, Donaldson MDC. Measured parental height in turner syndrome—a valuable but underused diagnostic tool. Eur J Pediatr. 2018;177:171–9.
2. Quigley CA, Crowe BJ, Anglin DG, Chipman JJ. Growth hormone and low dose estrogen in turner syndrome: results of a United States multi-center trial to near-final height. J Clin Endocrinol Metab. 2002;87:2033–41.
3. Seo GH, Kang E, Cho JH, Lee BH, Choi J-H, Kim G-H, Seo E-J, Yoo H-W. Turner syndrome presented with tall stature due to overdosage of the SHOX gene. Ann Pediatr Endocrinol Metab. 2015;20:110–3.
4. Oliveira CS, Alves C. The role of the SHOX gene in the pathophysiology of turner syndrome. Endocrinol Nutr. 2011;58:433–42.
5. Ross JL, Kowal K, Quigley CA, Blum WF, Cutler GB, Crowe B, Hovanes K, Elder FF, Zinn AR. The phenotype of short stature Homeobox gene (SHOX) deficiency in childhood: contrasting children with Leri-Weill Dyschondrosteosis and turner syndrome. J Pediatr. 2005;147:499–507.
6. Zhong Q, Layman LC. Genetic Considerations in the Patient with Turner Syndrome—45,X with or without Mosaicism. Fertil Steril. 2012;98:775–9.
7. Shankar RK, Backeljauw PF. Current best practice in the management of turner syndrome. Ther Adv Endocrinol Metab. 2018;9:33–40.
8. Atton G, Gordon K, Brice G, Keeley V, Riches K, Ostergaard P, Mortimer P, Mansour S. The lymphatic phenotype in turner syndrome: an evaluation of nineteen patients and literature review. Eur J Hum Genet. 2015;23:1634–9.
9. De Groote K, Demulier L, De Backer J, De Wolf D, De Schepper J, T'sjoen G, De Backer T. Arterial hypertension in turner syndrome: a review of the literature and a practical approach for diagnosis and treatment. J Hypertens. 2015;33:1342–51.
10. Evan L, Emilio Q, Zunqiu C, Jodi L, Michael S. Pilot study of blood pressure in girls with turner syndrome. Hypertension. 2016;68:133–6.
11. Becker B, Jospe N, Goldsmith LA. Melanocytic nevi in turner syndrome. Pediatr Dermatol. 1994;11:120–4.
12. Gibbs P, Brady BM, Gonzalez R, Robinson WA. Nevi and melanoma: lessons from Turner's syndrome. Dermatology (Basel). 2001;202:1–3.

13. Abir R, Fisch B, Nahum R, Orvieto R, Nitke S, Ben Rafael Z. Turner's syndrome and fertility: current status and possible putative prospects. Hum Reprod Update. 2001;7:603–10.
14. Bakalov VK, Cheng C, Zhou J, Bondy CA. X-chromosome gene dosage and the risk of diabetes in turner syndrome. J Clin Endocrinol Metabol. 2009;94:3289–96.
15. Collett-Solberg PF, Gallicchio CT, Da Coelho SSC Siqueira RA, De Alves STF, Guimarães MM (2011) Endocrine diseases, perspectives and care in turner syndrome. Arq Bras Endocrinol Metabol 55:550–558.
16. Feng J-G, Guo Y, Ma L-A, Xing J, Sun R-F, Zhu W. Prevalence of dermatologic manifestations and metabolic biomarkers in women with polycystic ovary syndrome in North China. J Cosmet Dermatol. 2018;17:511–7.
17. Ferriman D, Gallwey JD. Clinical assessment of body hair growth in women. J Clin Endocrinol Metab. 1961;21:1440–7.
18. Cook H, Brennan K, Azziz R. Reanalyzing the modified ferriman-gallwey score: is there a simpler method for assessing the extent of hirsutism? Fertil Steril. 2011;96:1266–1270.e1.
19. Aswini R, Jayapalan S. Modified Ferriman–Gallwey score in hirsutism and its association with metabolic syndrome. Int J Trichology. 2017;9:7–13.
20. Hatch R, Rosenfield RL, Kim MH, Tredway D. Hirsutism: implications, etiology, and management. Am J Obstet Gynecol. 1981;140:815–30.
21. Rosenfield RL. Clinical practice. Hirsutism. N Engl J Med. 2005;353:2578–88.
22. Coskun A, Ercan O, Arikan DC, Özer A, Kilinc M, Kiran G, Kostu B. Modified Ferriman–Gallwey hirsutism score and androgen levels in Turkish women. European Journal of Obstetrics and Gynecology and Reproductive Biology. 2011;154:167–71.
23. Escobar-Morreale HF, Carmina E, Dewailly D, et al. Epidemiology, diagnosis and management of hirsutism: a consensus statement by the androgen excess and polycystic ovary syndrome society. Hum Reprod Update. 2012;18:146–70.
24. Martin KA, Anderson RR, Chang RJ, Ehrmann DA, Lobo RA, Murad MH, Pugeat MM, Rosenfield RL. Evaluation and treatment of hirsutism in premenopausal women: an Endocrine Society clinical practice guideline. J Clin Endocrinol Metab. 2018;103:1233–57.
25. Mihailidis J, Dermesropian R, Taxel P, Luthra P, Grant-Kels JM. Endocrine evaluation of hirsutism. Int J Womens Dermatol. 2017;3:S6–S10.
26. Panidis D, Skiadopoulos S, Rousso D, Ioannides D, Panidou E. Association of acanthosis nigricans with insulin resistance in patients with polycystic ovary syndrome. Br J Dermatol. 1995;132:936–41.
27. Azziz R, Marin C, Hoq L, Badamgarav E, Song P. Health care-related economic burden of the polycystic ovary syndrome during the reproductive life span. J Clin Endocrinol Metab. 2005;90:4650–8.
28. Chuan SS, Chang RJ. Polycystic ovary syndrome and acne. Skin Therapy Lett. 2010;15:1–4.
29. Ju Q, Tao T, Hu T, Karadağ AS, Al-Khuzaei S, Chen W. Sex hormones and acne. Clin Dermatol. 2017;35:130–7.
30. Khezrian L, Yazdanfar A, Azizian Z, Hassani P, Feyzian M. The relationship between acne and other Hyperandrogenism signs. Journal of Skin and Stem Cell. 2016;3:e64187.
31. Sam S. Obesity and polycystic ovary syndrome. Obes Manag. 2007;3:69–73.
32. Boumosleh JM, Grundy SM, Phan J, Neeland IJ, Chang A, Vega GL. Metabolic concomitants of obese and nonobese women with features of polycystic ovarian syndrome. J Endocr Soc. 2017;1:1417–27.
33. Leondires MP, Berga SL. Role of GnRH drive in the pathophysiology of polycystic ovary syndrome. J Endocrinol Investig. 1998;21:476–85.
34. Chaudhari N, Dawalbhakta M, Nampoothiri L. GnRH dysregulation in polycystic ovarian syndrome (PCOS) is a manifestation of an altered neurotransmitter profile. Reprod Biol Endocrinol. 2018;16:37.
35. Johansson J, Stener-Victorin E. Polycystic ovary syndrome: effect and mechanisms of acupuncture for ovulation induction. Evid Based Complement Alternat Med. 2013; https://doi.org/10.1155/2013/762615.

36. Deswal R, Yadav A, Dang AS. Sex hormone binding globulin - an important biomarker for predicting PCOS risk: a systematic review and meta-analysis. Syst Biol Reprod Med. 2018;64:12–24.
37. Mehrabian F, Afghahi M. Can sex-hormone binding globulin considered as a predictor of response to pharmacological treatment in women with polycystic ovary syndrome? Int J Prev Med. 2013;4:1169–74.
38. Bremer AA. Polycystic ovary syndrome in the pediatric population. Metab Syndr Relat Disord. 2010;8:375–94.
39. Baskind NE, Balen AH. Hypothalamic-pituitary, ovarian and adrenal contributions to polycystic ovary syndrome. Best Pract Res Clin Obstet Gynaecol. 2016;37:80–97.
40. Dunaif A. Insulin resistance and the polycystic ovary syndrome: mechanism and implications for pathogenesis. Endocr Rev. 1997;18:774–800.
41. Yazıcı D, Sezer H. Insulin resistance, obesity and lipotoxicity. Adv Exp Med Biol. 2017;960:277–304.
42. Chen X, Jia X, Qiao J, Guan Y, Kang J. Adipokines in reproductive function: a link between obesity and polycystic ovary syndrome. J Mol Endocrinol. 2013;50:R21–37.
43. Dimitriadis GK, Kyrou I, Randeva HS. Polycystic ovary syndrome as a Proinflammatory state: the role of Adipokines. Curr Pharm Des. 2016;22:5535–46.
44. Legro RS, Arslanian SA, Ehrmann DA, Hoeger KM, Murad MH, Pasquali R, Welt CK. Diagnosis and treatment of polycystic ovary syndrome: an Endocrine Society clinical practice guideline. J Clin Endocrinol Metab. 2013;98:4565–92.
45. Ruiz-Olvera SF, Rajmil O, Sanchez-Curbelo J-R, Vinay J, Rodriguez-Espinosa J, Ruiz-Castañé E. Association of serum testosterone levels and testicular volume in adult patients. Andrologia. 2018;50:e12933.
46. Basaria S. Male hypogonadism. Lancet. 2014;383:1250–63.
47. Sakamoto H, Saito K, Ogawa Y, Yoshida H. Testicular volume measurements using Prader Orchidometer versus ultrasonography in patients with infertility. Urology. 2007;69:158–62.
48. Handelsman DJ, Staraj S. Testicular size: the effects of aging, malnutrition, and illness. J Androl. 1985;6:144–51.
49. Barrionuevo F, Burgos M, Jiménez R. Origin and function of embryonic Sertoli cells. Biomol Concepts. 2011;2:537–47.
50. Griswold MD. The central role of Sertoli cells in spermatogenesis. Semin Cell Dev Biol. 1998;9:411–6.
51. Shalet SM. Normal testicular function and spermatogenesis. Pediatr Blood Cancer. 2009;53:285–8.
52. Stocco C. Tissue physiology and pathology of aromatase. Steroids. 2012;77:27–35.
53. Vaucher L, Funaro MG, Mehta A, Mielnik A, Bolyakov A, Prossnitz ER, Schlegel PN, Paduch DA. Activation of GPER-1 estradiol receptor downregulates production of testosterone in isolated rat Leydig cells and adult human testis. PLoS One. 2014;9:e92425.
54. Demyashkin GA. Inhibin B in seminiferous tubules of human testes in normal spermatogenesis and in idiopathic infertility. Syst Biol Reprod Med. 2019;65:20–8.
55. Lin C-C, Huang WJS, Chen K-K. Measurement of testicular volume in smaller testes: how accurate is the conventional Orchidometer? J Androl. 2009;30:685–9.
56. Carlson HE. Approach to the patient with gynecomastia. J Clin Endocrinol Metab. 2011;96:15–21.
57. Meerkotter D. Gynaecomastia associated with highly active antiretroviral therapy (HAART). J Radiol Case Rep. 2010;4:34–40.
58. Ryan CS, Petkov VI, Adler RA. Osteoporosis in men: the value of laboratory testing. Osteoporos Int. 2011;22:1845–53.
59. Khosla S, Oursler MJ, Monroe DG. Estrogen and the skeleton. Trends Endocrinol Metab. 2012;23:576–81.
60. Szulc P, Claustrat B, Marchand F, Delmas PD. Increased risk of falls and increased bone resorption in elderly men with partial androgen deficiency: the MINOS study. J Clin Endocrinol Metabol. 2003;88:5240–7.

61. Rochira V, Kara E, Carani C. The endocrine role of estrogens on human male skeleton. Int J Endocrinol. 2015; https://doi.org/10.1155/2015/165215.
62. Skinner JW, Otzel DM, Bowser A, Nargi D, Agarwal S, Peterson MD, Zou B, Borst SE, Yarrow JF. Muscular responses to testosterone replacement vary by administration route: a systematic review and meta-analysis. J Cachexia Sarcopenia Muscle. 2018;9:465–81.
63. Brodsky IG, Balagopal P, Nair KS. Effects of testosterone replacement on muscle mass and muscle protein synthesis in hypogonadal men--a clinical research center study. J Clin Endocrinol Metab. 1996;81:3469–75.
64. Nieschlag E. Klinefelter Syndrome. Dtsch Arztebl Int. 2013;110:347–53.
65. Bonomi M, Rochira V, Pasquali D, Balercia G, Jannini EA, Ferlin A. Klinefelter syndrome (KS): genetics, clinical phenotype and hypogonadism. J Endocrinol Investig. 2017;40: 123–34.
66. Urysiak-Czubatka I, Kmieć ML, Broniarczyk-Dyła G. Assessment of the usefulness of dihydrotestosterone in the diagnostics of patients with androgenetic alopecia. Postepy Dermatol Alergol. 2014;31:207–15.
67. El Kassar N, Hetet G, Brière J, Grandchamp B. X-chromosome inactivation in healthy females: incidence of excessive lyonization with age and comparison of assays involving DNA methylation and transcript polymorphisms. Clin Chem. 1998;44:61–7.
68. Groth KA, Skakkebæk A, Høst C, Gravholt CH, Bojesen A. Klinefelter syndrome—a clinical update. J Clin Endocrinol Metab. 2013;98:20–30.
69. Terribile M, Stizzo M, Manfredi C, Quattrone C, Bottone F, Giordano RD, Bellastella G, Arcaniolo D, De Sio M. 46,XX Testicular Disorder of Sex Development (DSD): A Case Report and Systematic Review. Medicina. 2019; https://doi.org/10.3390/medicina55070371.
70. Li T-F, Wu Q-Y, Zhang C, Li W-W, Zhou Q, Jiang W-J, Cui Y-X, Xia X-Y, Shi Y-C. 46,XX testicular disorder of sexual development with SRY-negative caused by some unidentified mechanisms: a case report and review of the literature. BMC Urol. 2014;14:104.
71. Huang AJ, Moore EE, Boyko EJ, Scholes D, Lin F, Vittinghoff E, Fihn SD. Vaginal symptoms in postmenopausal women: self-reported severity, natural history, and risk factors. Menopause. 2010;17:121–6.
72. Waetjen LE, Crawford SL, Chang P, Reed BD, Hess R, Avis NE, Harlow SD, Greendale GA, Dugan SA, Gold EB. Factors associated with developing vaginal dryness symptoms in women transitioning through menopause: a longitudinal study. Menopause. 2018;25:1094–104.
73. Santoro N, Epperson CN, Mathews SB. Menopausal symptoms and their management. Endocrinol Metab Clin N Am. 2015;44:497–515.
74. Nair PA. Dermatosis associated with menopause. J Midlife Health. 2014;5:168–75.
75. Shah M, Karena Z, Patel SV, Parmar N, Singh PK, Sharma A. Treatment of vaginal atrophy with vaginal estrogen cream in menopausal Indian women. Oman Med J. 2017;32:15–9.
76. Mac Bride MB, Rhodes DJ, Shuster LT. Vulvovaginal atrophy. Mayo Clin Proc. 2010;85:87–94.
77. Finkelstein JS, Brockwell SE, Mehta V, et al. Bone mineral density changes during the menopause transition in a multiethnic cohort of women. J Clin Endocrinol Metab. 2008;93: 861–8.
78. Manolagas SC, O'Brien CA, Almeida M. The role of estrogen and androgen receptors in bone health and disease. Nat Rev Endocrinol. 2013;9:699–712.
79. Wang J, Zhang W, Yu C, Zhang X, Zhang H, Guan Q, Zhao J, Xu J. Follicle-stimulating hormone increases the risk of postmenopausal osteoporosis by stimulating osteoclast differentiation. PLoS One. 2015; https://doi.org/10.1371/journal.pone.0134986.
80. Chin K-Y. The relationship between follicle-stimulating hormone and bone health: alternative explanation for bone loss beyond Oestrogen? Int J Med Sci. 2018;15:1373–83.
81. Barbat-Artigas S, Aubertin-Leheudre M. Menopausal transition and fat distribution. Menopause. 2013;20:370.
82. Lovejoy J, Champagne C, de Jonge L, Xie H, Smith S. Increased visceral fat and decreased energy expenditure during the menopausal transition. Int J Obes. 2008;32:949–58.

83. Leanne H, Rajarshi B, Belén R, et al. Menopausal Status and Abdominal Obesity Are Significant Determinants of Hepatic Lipid Metabolism in Women. Journal of the American Heart Association. 4:e002258.
84. Donato GB, Fuchs SC, Oppermann K, Bastos C, Spritzer PM. Association between menopause status and central adiposity measured at different cutoffs of waist circumference and waist-to-hip ratio. Menopause. 2006;13:280–5.
85. Kozakowski J, Gietka-Czernel M, Leszczyńska D, Majos A. Obesity in menopause – our negligence or an unfortunate inevitability? Prz Menopauzalny. 2017;16:61–5.
86. Freedman RR. Pathophysiology and treatment of menopausal hot flashes. Semin Reprod Med. 2005;23:117–25.
87. Morrow PKH, Mattair DN, Hortobagyi GN. Hot flashes: a review of pathophysiology and treatment modalities. Oncologist. 2011;16:1658–64.
88. Freeman EW, Sammel MD, Sanders RJ. Risk of long term hot flashes after natural menopause: evidence from the penn ovarian aging cohort. Menopause. 2014;21:924–32.
89. Gordon M, Donald L, Emanuele M, Ann M. Hot flashes in patients with hypogonadism and low serum gon-adotropin levels. Endocr Pract. 2003;9:119–23.
90. Szafran H, Smielak-Korombel W. The role of estrogens in hormonal regulation of lipid metabolism in women. Przeglad lekarski. 1998;55:266–70.
91. Kumar S, Shah C, Oommen ER. Study of cardiovascular risk factors in pre and postmenopausal women. Int J Pharma Sci Res. 2012;3:560–70.
92. Smith EP, Boyd J, Frank GR, Takahashi H, Cohen RM, Specker B, Williams TC, Lubahn DB, Korach KS. Estrogen resistance caused by a mutation in the estrogen-receptor gene in a man. N Engl J Med. 1994;331:1056–61.
93. Bernard V, Kherra S, Francou B, et al. Familial multiplicity of estrogen insensitivity associated with a loss-of-function ESR1 mutation. J Clin Endocrinol Metab. 2016;102:93–9.
94. Quaynor SD, Stradtman EW, Kim H-G, Shen Y, Chorich LP, Schreihofer DA, Layman LC. Delayed puberty and estrogen resistance in a woman with estrogen receptor α variant. N Engl J Med. 2013;369:164–71.
95. Simm PJ, Bajpai A, Russo VC, Werther GA. Estrogens and growth. Pediatr Endocrinol Rev. 2008;6:32–41.
96. Rodd C, Jourdain N, Alini M. Action of estradiol on epiphyseal growth plate chondrocytes. Calcif Tissue Int. 2004;75:214–24.
97. Nilsson O, Marino R, De Luca F, Phillip M, Baron J. Endocrine regulation of the growth plate. Horm Res. 2005;64:157–65.
98. Hewitt SC, Korach KS. Estrogen receptors: new directions in the new millennium. Endocr Rev. 2018;39:664–75.
99. Lang-Muritano M, Sproll P, Wyss S, Kolly A, Hürlimann R, Konrad D, Biason-Lauber A. Early-onset complete ovarian failure and lack of puberty in a woman with mutated estrogen receptor β (ESR2). J Clin Endocrinol Metab. 2018;103:3748–56.
100. Yang P, Liu X, Gao J, Qu S, Zhang M. Complete androgen insensitivity syndrome in a young woman with metabolic disorder and diabetes: a case report. Medicine (Baltimore). 2018;97:e11353.
101. Batista RL, Costa EMF, De Rodrigues AS, et al. Androgen insensitivity syndrome: a review. Archives of Endocrinology and Metabolism. 2018;62:227–35.
102. Mendoza N, Motos MA. Androgen insensitivity syndrome. Gynecol Endocrinol. 2013;29:1–5.
103. Mongan NP, Tadokoro-Cuccaro R, Bunch T, Hughes IA. Androgen insensitivity syndrome. Best Pract Res Clin Endocrinol Metab. 2015;29:569–80.
104. Hughes IA, Davies JD, Bunch TI, Pasterski V, Mastroyannopoulou K, MacDougall J. Androgen insensitivity syndrome. Lancet. 2012;380:1419–28.
105. Nazzaro G, Genovese G, Brena M, Passoni E, Tadini G. Aberrant breast tissue in complete androgen insensitivity syndrome. Clin Exp Dermatol. 2018;43:491–3.
106. Tadokoro-Cuccaro R, Hughes IA. Androgen insensitivity syndrome. Curr Opin Endocrinol Diabetes Obes. 2014;21:499.

107. T'Sjoen G, De Cuypere G, Monstrey S, Hoebeke P, Freedman FK, Appari M, Holterhus P-M, Van Borsel J, Cools M. Male gender identity in complete androgen insensitivity syndrome. Arch Sex Behav. 2011;40:635–8.
108. Souhail R, Amine S, Nadia A, Tarik K, Khalid EK, Abdellatif K, Ahmed IA. Complete androgen insensitivity syndrome or testicular feminization: review of literature based on a case report. Pan Afr Med J. 2016; https://doi.org/10.11604/pamj.2016.25.199.10758.
109. Quigley CA, de Bellis A, Marschke KB, El-Awady MK, Wilson EM, French FS. Androgen receptor defects: historical, clinical, and molecular perspectives. Endocr Rev. 1995;16:271–321.

Signs in Disorders of Lipid Metabolism and Obesity

7

Learning Objectives

At the end of this chapter, you will be able to:

1. Understand the pathophysiologic basis for the cutaneous manifestations of lipid disorders
2. Understand lipid metabolism and how various enzyme defects account for the clinical and biochemical phenotypes seen in various causes of dyslipidemia
3. Recognize the pathophysiologic basis for the clinical manifestations of monogenic causes of obesity (congenital leptin and POMC deficiencies)

7.1 Signs in Disorders of Lipid Metabolism

7.1.1 Corneal Arcus

Clinical Features

Corneal arcus (CA) is a circumferential deposition of lipids in the cornea and appears as whitish-gray deposits around the cornea with a predilection for the superior and inferior limbus of the cornea. It eventually progresses to involve the entire peripheral rim of the cornea [1].

CA is widely accepted as a typical sign of the aging process, although it might signify the presence of dyslipidemia [2, 3]. A population-based prospective study involving more than 3600 subjects in Asia assessed the association of CA with cardiovascular disease (CVD) events.

The authors prospectively evaluated CVD events after an initial confirmation of the presence of CA. After adjusting for baseline traditional risk factors, CA was associated with a clinically significant increased odds ratio (OR) of 1.52 [1.07 to 2.16] for incident CVD [4].

© Springer Nature Switzerland AG 2020
A. Manni, A. Quarde, *Endocrine Pathophysiology*,
https://doi.org/10.1007/978-3-030-49872-6_7

Pathophysiology
- Unlike atherosclerosis, CA is not due to endothelial dysfunction. There is no evidence of foam cells (lipid-filled macrophages), which implies there is an alternative mechanism explaining the characteristic histopathologic findings in CA [5].
- There is a mismatch between the influx and efflux of lipids in the cornea, with the balance tilted toward excessive lipid influx [5]. Indeed, the 12 o'clock position of the peripheral cornea tends to have a higher density of deposited lipids since the superior corneal limbus is more vascularized compared to the rest of the peripheral cornea [6].
- Other less validated reasons for CA include an immune-mediated reaction to either age-related ocular degeneration or inflammation [7].

7.1.2   Xanthomas and Xanthelasma

Clinical Features
Xanthomas represent localized regions of accumulated lipids in the skin, subcutaneous tissues, and tendons [8, 9]. They may be plaque-like, papular, or nodular lesions, depending on the morphologic subtype [8, 10].

Tuberous xanthomas are characteristically distributed over pressure points (sites of trauma) such as the elbows and knees [9]. They are firm, yellowish-red papulonodular skin lesions [11], which vary in size from a few millimeters [12] to massive xanthomas [13]. Tuberous xanthomas occur in patients with familial hypercholesterolemia (type 2A hyperlipoproteinemia) [14, 15] and familial dysbetalipoproteinemia (type 3 hyperlipoproteinemia) [16].

Eruptive xanthomas (*EX*), on the other hand, tend to present in patients with type 1, 4, or 5 hyperlipoproteinemia [16]. EX has a reported prevalence of 1.7 for every 10,000 patients [17]. Secondary causes of EX include diabetes mellitus, hypothyroidism, alcohol use, cholestasis, and estrogens [18].

- They may vary from yellowish-orange to reddish-brown papules with a circumferential erythematous hue. EX are usually located over extensor surfaces of the extremities but may occur in flexural areas and the trunk.
- EX lesions exhibit the Koebner phenomenon, i.e., new lesions develop along the sites of cutaneous trauma or irritation [19].

Palmar xanthomas (PX) appear as yellowish-orange macules with a predilection for the palmar creases [20]. They are pathognomonic for type 3 hyperlipoproteinemia (familial dysbetalipoproteinemia) [16] and may, on rare occasions, occur in patients with familial hypercholesterolemia [21]. PX should be distinguished from planar xanthomas, which are whitish plaques and tend to extend beyond the confines of the palmar creases [20]. Palmar xanthomas are classically referred to as xanthoma striatum palmare [22].

Xanthelasmas are the most common *cutaneous xanthoma* [23] and are distributed over the inner canthus of the upper eyelids [24, 25]. The lesions are soft, yellowish plaques and may be observed in other sites apart from the periorbital region, such as the axilla, neck, and trunk [26]. In a large prospective cohort study involving more than 12,000 subjects [3], investigators were able to demonstrate that xanthelasmas were independently associated with ischemic heart disease after controlling for some CVD risk factors such as elevated plasma cholesterol and triglycerides [3].

Pathophysiology
Unlike the underlying pathophysiology of corneal arcus [5], the formation of xanthomas is similar to that of atherosclerotic plaques. Leakage of lipids from cutaneous vessels results in excessive lipid deposition in the skin [27]. Dermal lipids are then phagocytosed by macrophages, which evolve into foam cells (lipid-laden macrophages), a critical step in the formation of xanthomas. Xanthomas, in effect, represent oxidized LDL cholesterol particles present in the skin and connective tissue [5, 8, 10, 28].

7.1.3 Skin Crease (Frank's Sign)

Clinical Features
Frank's sign is a diagonal wrinkle involving the skin of the ear lobe [29]. This presumed dermatologic manifestation of atherosclerotic disease was first reported by Dr. Sanders Frank in 1973, in a letter titled "Aural Sign of Coronary-Artery Disease," published in the *New Journal of Medicine* (NEJM) [30].

It is thought to increase with age and is associated with some cardiovascular risk factors [5]. There is conflicting evidence in the literature regarding the association of Frank's sign with atherosclerotic disease [31, 32]. The association of Frank's sign with atherosclerotic disease might, however, not necessarily imply a direct causal relationship.

Pathophysiology
Dyslipidemia-induced microangiopathy leading to ischemia and eventual breakdown of elastic fibers accounts for the skin changes seen with Frank's sign [31]. The reason for the predilection of this cutaneous lesion for the ear lobe is, however, unclear.

7.1.4 Lipemia Retinalis

Clinical Features
It is a rare fundoscopic examination finding in patients with markedly elevated serum triglycerides [33]. The vessels in the posterior pole and peripheral aspect of the retina develop a creamy white appearance that can be visualized on the fundoscopic exam [34–36]. Some patients may have deterioration of visual acuity, which improves upon initiation of anti-lipidemic therapy [33].

Pathophysiology

The creamy appearance of the retinal vessels has been attributed to the high content of triglyceride-rich chylomicrons reflecting direct light from the ophthalmoscope [37].

 Pathophysiology Pearl

What are lipoproteins?

Lipoproteins: They are a complex composition of cholesterol esters and triacylglycerols in a dense lipid core, with a circumferential rim of free cholesterol, apolipoproteins, and phospholipids. This intricate configuration allows water-insoluble cholesterol and triacylglycerols to be ferried through the circulatory system to their target tissues [38, 39]. The classification of lipoproteins depends on their *size*, *lipid composition*, and specific *apolipoproteins* subtype. There are various lipoproteins, including low-density lipoprotein (LDL), high-density lipoproteins (HDL), very low-density lipoproteins (VLDL), intermediate-density lipoproteins (IDL), and chylomicrons [40].

Apoproteins/apolipoproteins: These complex proteins present on the surface of lipoproteins play critical roles in lipoprotein physiology by providing structural integrity to lipoproteins, modulating lipoprotein-related enzymatic action, and serving as ligands for various lipoproteins at specific target tissues [41].

 Pathophysiology Pearl

Lipoprotein Metabolism

Lipoprotein metabolism aims to transfer dietary sources of triglycerides to both muscle and adipose tissue for energy metabolism and storage, respectively. It also facilitates the cycling of cholesterol between the liver and peripheral tissues, a process critical for the formation of steroid hormones, cell membranes, and bile acids [42].

Step 1: Bile salts emulsify fat globules into smaller fatty droplets that contain triglycerides (TAGs) and cholesterol esters (CEs). Dietary triglycerides are then hydrolyzed into free fatty acids (FFAs) and monoacylglycerol (MAG) in the intestinal lumen by pancreatic lipases. This initial step enables the eventual transfer of TAGs from the intestinal lumen into the circulatory system. The products of hydrolysis of TAGs, i.e., FFAs and MAG, are then repackaged into micelles, which then diffuse into the cytosol of the enterocyte [42, 43]. Once in the enterocyte, FFAs and MAG are then resynthesized into TAGs in preparation for delivery to the circulatory system. TAGs, cholesterol esters, cholesterol, and apolipoprotein B-48 (Apo B-48) are then packaged into chylomicrons in the enterocyte [44]. This concludes the formation of the first lipoprotein in the exogenous lipoprotein pathway [45].

Step 2: Chylomicrons enter systemic circulation via the thoracic duct, thus bypassing the portal circulation [43, 46].

Once in the systemic circulation, HDL transfers apolipoprotein CII (Apo-CII) and apolipoprotein E (Apo-E) to chylomicrons. Apo-E allows the binding of lipoproteins to specific LDL receptors or LDL-like receptors present in various tissues (liver and adrenal cortex). Apo-CII, on the other hand, is critical in activating the lipoprotein lipase, present on the capillary endothelium [47].

Step 3: Chylomicrons reach adipose tissue and muscle, where lipoprotein lipase (produced by adipocytes and muscle cells) present on the endothelial lining of capillaries hydrolyzes TAGs into FFAs and monoacylglycerol. FFAs are then taken up by adipocytes and muscle cells for energy metabolism [42]. Chylomicron remnants, which are formed after this step, then release the previously acquired apo-CII, which was needed for lipoprotein lipase activity, back to HDL [48]. This concludes the exogenous lipoprotein pathway, which facilitates the transfer of dietary sources of fatty acids from the intestine to muscle and adipose tissue, for both storage and metabolism [49].

Step 4: Chylomicron remnants, which contain mostly cholesterol and cholesterol esters, bind to the hepatic LDL receptor and are transported into the liver [50].

Step 5: Once in the liver, TAGs, cholesterol esters, and Apo-B100 are repackaged into VLDL. VLDL in circulation, just like chylomicrons, receives Apo-E and Apo-CII from HDL. VLDL is transported to adipose tissue and the muscle, where, again, lipoprotein lipase facilitates the hydrolysis of TAGs into FFAs and monoacylglycerol. FFAs can then be stored in fatty tissue or used for energy metabolism by muscle. The loss of TAGs from VLDL results in the formation of intermediate-density lipoproteins (IDL) or VLDL remnants. Again, Apo-CII will be released back to HDL after the formation of IDL [47, 51].

Step 6: IDL in circulation, with its surface-bound Apo-E, has an affinity for tissues with LDL or LDL-like receptors. IDL binds to the hepatic LDL receptor, where it is taken up by the liver for further processing. Apo-B100 and cholesterol esters are then repackaged into a new lipoprotein called LDL [47].

Step 7: LDL binds LDL-like receptors in the gonads for gonadal steroidogenesis [52] and the adrenal cortex for adrenal steroidogenesis [53, 54]. LDL can also bind LDL receptors present in muscle and adipose tissue, where it can be taken up for further processing. Ultimately, LDL tracks back to the liver to conclude the endogenous lipoprotein pathway, whose primary purpose is to transfer cholesterol and TAGs from the liver to peripheral tissues [55]. Figure 7.1 depicts critical steps in the lipoprotein synthesis pathway.

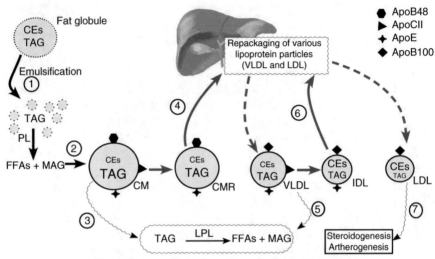

Target tissues : Skeletal muscle and adipose tissue

Fig. 7.1 Exogenous and endogenous lipoprotein pathway. Emulsification of fat globules into tiny fat droplets by bile (step 1) [42–44] facilitates the hydrolysis of triacylglycerides (TAGs) into free fatty acids (FFAs) and monoacylglycerol (MAG) by pancreatic lipase (PL) in the intestinal lumen. Chylomicron (CM) formed from repackaged TAG, cholesterol esters (CEs), and various apoproteins (step 2) [43, 46, 47] are delivered to target tissues where TAG is hydrolyzed by lipoprotein lipase (LPL) (step 3) [42, 48, 49]. Chylomicron remnants (CMR) are transported to the liver for further processing (step 4) [50]. VLDL released from the liver is destined for adipose tissue and skeletal muscle, where stores of TAG are released for hydrolysis by LPL (step 5) [47, 51]. IDL formed after VLDL processing in target tissues is destined for the liver (step 6) [47]. LDL, a cholesterol ester (CE)-rich lipoprotein, is critical in steroidogenesis in various tissues and plays a central role in atherogenesis (step 7) [53–55]. (Redrawn and modified from Ramasamy [42])

☀ Pathophysiology Pearl

Reverse Cholesterol Transport Pathway

HDL is responsible for transferring cholesterol and triglycerides from peripheral tissues back to the liver [56] and finally into the intestine for excretion [57] (Fig. 7.2).

💡 Questions You Might Be Asked on Clinical Rounds

What are the underlying pathophysiologic mechanisms for the various types of dyslipidemia?

Type 1 Hyperlipoproteinemia

Deficiencies of either lipoprotein lipase (LPL) [63] or apolipoprotein CII (Apo-CII) have been reported [45]. These defects result in an elevated level of triglyceride-rich chylomicrons. Clinical features include recurrent pancreatitis, lipemia retinalis, tubero-eruptive xanthomas, and hepatosplenomegaly [64].

Sources of cholesterol

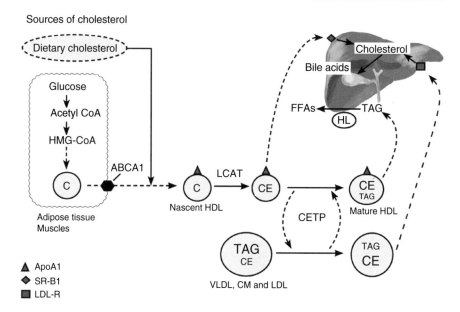

Fig. 7.2 Schematic representation of reverse cholesterol transport pathway. Free cholesterol from extrahepatic tissues (muscles and adipose tissue) is transferred to ApoA-1 to form the nascent HDL particle; this process is facilitated by ATP-binding cassette transporter A1 (ABCA1) present on the cell membrane of extrahepatic tissues (muscles, adipose tissue, and intestine). Cholesterol (C) is then converted to cholesterol esters by Lecithin-cholesterol acyltransferase (LCAT), which is critical in the formation of mature HDL [47]. Cholesterol ester transfer protein (CETP) is essential in the transfer of cholesterol esters and triglycerides between other circulating lipoproteins (chylomicrons, VLDL, LDL) and HDL. CETP transfers CEs from HDL to other lipoproteins and carries TAGs from these lipoproteins back to the mature HDL particle. HDL, therefore, becomes rich in TAGs at the expense of CEs [58]. HDL binds to the hepatic scavenger SR-B1 receptor, where it releases its cholesterol esters without being internalized by the liver. It then returns to circulation as a smaller HDL particle, to repeat the process of cholesterol and triglyceride acquisition [59, 60]. HDL may also be hydrolyzed by hepatic lipase (HL) into FFAs, converting it back to a smaller HDL particle, which can then be recycled in the process of cholesterol acquisition. HDL can also bind the hepatic LDL-R receptor [61], a process that facilitates the release of cholesterol to the liver for bile acid synthesis [62]. (Redrawn and modified from Ramasamy [42])

We will refer readers to step 3 of the lipoprotein synthesis pathway reviewed in Fig. 7.1. Note the importance of Apo CII and lipoprotein lipase in the hydrolysis of triglyceride-laden chylomicrons.

Type 2A Hyperlipoproteinemia (Familial Hypercholesterolemia)

Mutations in the LDL receptor (LDL-R) and apolipoprotein B (ApoB) genes have been reported [65], with mutations of the LDL-R accounting for 85–90% of cases [66]. Activating mutations in proprotein convertase subtilisin kexin type 9 (PCSK9), an enzyme complex involved in the recycling of the LDL-R, limits the life span of the LDL-R and is responsible for a small subset of cases of type 2A hyperlipoproteinemia [66].

There is an elevated level of total cholesterol and LDL. HDL and TAGs are usually normal [66].

Clinical features include corneal arcus, xanthelasma, or tuberous xanthomas [66].

Type 2B Hyperlipoproteinemia (Familial Combined Hyperlipidemia)

It is the most common genetic cause of dyslipidemia in the general population. The primary defect in type 2B hyperlipidemia is yet to be elucidated [67]; it, however, leads to excessive production of VLDL (triglyceride-laden lipoprotein) [68] and LDL [69, 70].

This clinical phenotype fits the typical "atherogenic lipid triad," which consists of an elevated serum concentration of small dense LDL with high TAGs, high apolipoprotein B, and reduced HDL [68]. Physical findings suggestive of dyslipidemia are uncommon in familial combined hyperlipidemia [71]. It is worthy to note that the most frequent cause of dyslipidemia in the general population seldom has any of the physical manifestations we discussed earlier in this chapter.

Type 3 Hyperlipoproteinemia (Dysbetalipoproteinemia)

Elevated VLDL remnants (IDL) and chylomicrons account for the high levels of both total cholesterol and triglycerides in these patients [72]. There is a defect in the processing of chylomicrons and VLDL by the liver, which results in an increased circulating half-life of VLDL and chylomicrons. CETP, therefore, has an opportunity to transfer more cholesterol esters from HDL to CM and VLDL due to the high levels of the latter two lipoproteins in circulation. Elevated concentrations of these abnormal lipoproteins result in high blood cholesterol-triglyceride ratio [72].

Type 4 Hyperlipoproteinemia (Simple Hypertriglyceridemia)

An isolated elevation of VLDL characterizes simple hypertriglyceridemia. Unlike the monogenic inheritance pattern of familial hypercholesterolemia, type 4 hyperlipoproteinemia is instead mostly polygenic in its etiology [71]. There is an elevated level of mainly VLDL-derived plasma triglycerides [71] and concomitant lowering of HDL cholesterol [73].

Clinical features include eruptive xanthomas, lipemia retinalis, and hepatosplenomegaly [71]. Type 4 hyperlipoproteinemia seldom causes acute pancreatitis except during specific metabolic stresses, when the type 4 phenotype can change to a type 5 phenotype with both increased VLDL and chylomicrons [71].

This form of hyperlipoproteinemia is sometimes called *diabetic dyslipidemia* as it is frequently encountered in people with type 2 diabetes mellitus (T2DM) and is considered part of the metabolic (insulin resistance) syndrome [73]. It is also associated with cardiovascular disease [74] and nonalcoholic fatty liver disease [75].

Type 5 Hyperlipoproteinemia

The etiology is multifactorial, including genetic mutations that result in altered triglyceride metabolism. Acquired factors such as alcohol, uncontrolled diabetes, steroids, estrogens, and medications play contributory roles in type 5 hyperlipoproteinemia. It is characterized by VLDL and chylomicron elevation, which results in an elevation of both triglycerides and total cholesterol [76].

The clinical features are similar to those of type 1 hyperlipoproteinemia [71]. Unlike familial hyperchylomicronemia, patients with type 5 hyperlipoproteinemia are at risk for cardiovascular disease [77–79].

There is evidence that although large chylomicrons are unable to penetrate the vasculature, VLDL and smaller remnants of chylomicrons can disrupt the integrity of the vascular endothelium. This sets off an inflammatory cascade that culminates in significant atherogenesis [80]. A useful mnemonic for remembering the features of this type of dyslipidemia is 1 + 4 = 5 because it has the combined features of types 1 and 4 hyperlipoproteinemia.

Tangier Disease

Tangier disease is named after the island in Chesapeake Bay, from which the first reported cases hailed [81]. It is caused by a genetic mutation in the ATP-binding cassette transporter A1 (ABCA1) gene, a gene that encodes the critical regulatory membrane transporter ABCA1. ABCA1 mediates the transfer of free cholesterol from extrahepatic tissues to apoA-1, to form the nascent HDL particle [82].

It is a severe form of "hypolipoproteinemia," which affects HDL metabolism. Patients have very low serum HDL and low total cholesterol with normal or even high triglycerides [82]. The clinical features include yellowish-orange discoloration of the tonsils, tonsillar enlargement, hepatosplenomegaly, and peripheral neuropathy [81].

The defect in ABCA1-mediated mobilization of peripheral cholesterol leads to the accumulation of lipids in various tissues, including the spleen, nerves, skin, and lymphoid tissue. Indeed, the accumulation of lipids in neurons leads to their devitalization and eventual demyelination.

Familial LCAT Deficiency

Lecithin-cholesterol acyltransferase is a regulatory enzyme required for the esterification of peripherally acquired free cholesterol into cholesterol esters in the nascent HDL particle [83]. It is a rare condition with about 100 case reports to date [84].

Familial LCAT deficiency is due to mutations in the LCAT gene, which results in reduced esterification of free cholesterol into cholesterol esters. Patients with LCAT deficiency, therefore, have a high free cholesterol to esterified cholesterol ratio [85, 86].

Subjects with partial LCAT deficiency classically present with extensive corneal opacification that is often referred to as *fish-eye disease* (FED). Complete LCAT deficiency is composed of a triad of *corneal opacification (FED), anemia, and renal dysfunction* [87].

A summary of the various clinical phenotypes of hyperlipoproteinemias is based on Dr. Donald S. Fredrickson's classification, which was first

Table 7.1 Fredrickson classification of hyperlipoproteinemias

Type	Primary hyperlipidemia classification	Elevated lipoprotein
1	Familial hyperchylomicronemia syndrome	Chylomicrons [64]
2A	Familial hypercholesterolemia	LDL [66]
2B	Familial combined hypercholesterolemia	LDL, VLDL [69]
3	Familial dysbetalipoproteinemia	IDL [70, 72]
4	Simple hypertriglyceridemia	VLDL [71]
5	Familial hypertriglyceridemia	Chylomicrons, VLDL [76]

Adapted from references [64, 66, 69–72, 76]

published in the journal *Circulation* in 1965 [88]. The classification system is an oversimplification of the defects in lipoprotein metabolism but is a good starting point in terms of appreciating the various forms of hyperlipoproteinemias (Table 7.1).

Why do patients with hypertriglyceridemia develop acute pancreatitis? [89]

1. Pancreatic lipases hydrolyze elevated triglycerides present in the capillaries of the pancreas into FFAs and MAGs. Free fatty acids bind to serum calcium and cause direct damage to capillaries. This sets off a cascade of inflammatory reactions, which leads to the formation of multiple microthrombi that subsequently clogs up capillaries and contributes to ischemia [90].
2. High levels of circulating serum chylomicrons cause extensive sludging of blood in the pancreatic capillaries, which leads to pancreatic ischemia and acidemia [90].
3. Also, FFAs activate trypsinogen, a critical step that finally initiates pancreatitis [90].

7.2 Congenital Leptin Deficiency

7.2.1 Obesity

Clinical Features
Congenital leptin deficiency is associated with significant early-onset obesity [91]. Patients exhibit a somewhat ravenous food-seeking behavior and, as such, present with extreme obesity at a very young age [92].

Pathophysiology
1. Accumulation of fat mass due to excess caloric intake accounts for the obesity observed in patients with congenital leptin deficiency [93]. Leptin, a hormone secreted by *white adipose tissue*, is involved in triggering satiety through the central anorexigenic pathway [91]. Leptin binds to leptin receptors present on proopiomelanocortin (POMC) processing neurons in the arcuate nucleus of the hypothalamus to cause satiety [94]. Congenital leptin deficiency, therefore, causes hyperphagia and promotes excess weight gain [91].

2. Leptin also increases energy expenditure by potentiating sympathetic nerve activity in *brown adipose tissue*, a process which results in increased thermogenesis. Reduced energy expenditure, which occurs as a consequence of leptin deficiency, contributes to obesity [95].

 Questions You Might Be Asked on Clinical Rounds

What is the genetic basis of congenital leptin deficiency?
    The majority of patients with congenital leptin deficiency were conceived in consanguineous relationships [96]. It occurs as a result of a genetic mutation in the leptin receptor (LEPR) gene; thus, a defective protein is transcribed and translated [92].
    What are the other endocrine effects of leptin?

1. *Hypothalamic-pituitary-thyroidal axis*: Leptin regulates the release of thyroid-stimulating hormone (TSH) [97]. Central hypothyroidism occurs due to leptin-mediated signaling defects in the hypothalamic-pituitary-thyroid axis. Indeed, the amelioration of hypothyroidism occurs after optimal leptin replacement therapy [98].
2. *Hypothalamic-pituitary-gonadal axis*: Leptin regulates the release of gonadotropin-releasing hormone (GnRH) [95]. Patients with congenital leptin deficiency are hypogonadal due to defective GnRH release [97].

7.3   Proopiomelanocortin (POMC) Deficiency

7.3.1   Triad of Obesity, Adrenal Insufficiency, and Reddish Hair

Clinical Features
Early-onset obesity was reported as a clinical finding in the first case of POMC deficiency. Other clinical findings in this recently discovered monogenic cause of obesity included reddish pigmentation of body hair and features of central adrenal insufficiency [99]. Multiple case reports have been published since the index case [100–103].

Pathophysiology
Patients with POMC deficiency have a mutation in the POMC gene. POMC serves as a prohormone from which ACTH, α-MSH, and other anterior pituitary peptide hormones are derived [104].

1. Hyperphagia occurs due to signaling defects in the hypothalamic leptin-melanocortin anorexigenic pathway due to an absence of POMC [105].
2. The absence of melanocyte-stimulating hormone accounts for the hypopigmented skin and reddish hair seen in patients with this disorder [105]. α-MSH

mediates skin pigmentation by binding to the melanocortin type 1 receptor (MC1-R) present on skin melanocytes [106].
3. The absence of ACTH results in central adrenal insufficiency [105]. Under physiologic conditions, ACTH binds to melanocortin type 2 receptors in the adrenal cortex to facilitate glucocorticoid synthesis [107].

 Pathophysiology Pearl

POMC and the Anorexigenic (Satiety) Pathway

- POMC processing occurs in the arcuate nucleus of the hypothalamus, pituitary, and other parts of the brain. POMC is transcribed into a large polypeptide that undergoes proteolysis by the prohormone convertase 1 enzyme, to form ACTH and β-lipoprotein. β-Lipoprotein is subsequently converted into α-MSH and β-endorphin, respectively, by prohormone convertase 2 [108]. See Fig. 3.2.
- POMC then binds to melanocortin-4 receptors of the hypothalamus to trigger satiety (anorexigenic pathway) [109].

 Questions You Might Be Asked on Clinical Rounds

How do craniopharyngiomas cause hypothalamic obesity?

Craniopharyngiomas are benign tumors typically located in the sellar or parasellar regions. Treatment options for lesions located in the hypothalamus include surgical resection and radiation therapy [110].

Patients invariably develop hyperphagia and obesity because of tumor location or surgical treatment. Disruption of hypothalamic tracts, e.g., POMC signaling anorexigenic pathways, explains in part the onset of hyperphagia in these patients [111, 112].

What are the other clinical features seen in patients with POMC deficiency? (Table 7.2)

Table 7.2 Clinical features of POMC deficiency and their underlying mechanisms

Clinical features	Mechanism
Hypopigmented skin	Defects in MSH-mediated melanocyte activation [102]
Hypogonadotropic hypogonadism	Defects in POMC-mediated signaling of GnRH release [102]
Central hypothyroidism	Defects in POMC-mediated signaling of TRH release [102]
Hyponatremia	Increased ADH secretion in the setting of central hypocortisolemia. Elevated CRH is a secretagogue for antidiuretic hormone [102]

CRH corticotropin-releasing hormone
Adapted from Çetinkaya et al. [102]

7.4 Lipodystrophy Syndromes

7.4.1 Atrophy of Adipose Tissue

Clinical Features
The distribution of adipose tissue atrophy is variable in patients with lipodystrophy syndromes and is dependent on the underlying cause [113, 114] (Table 7.3).

Pathophysiology
1. Several enzymes involved in triglyceride and phospholipid metabolism are impaired (*Congenital generalized lipodystrophy*). These complex enzyme defects impair both the synthesis of phospholipids in adipose tissue and adipocyte differentiation.
2. Autoimmune-mediated panniculitis (inflammation of subcutaneous tissue).
3. Protease inhibitors impair various factors involved in adipose tissue synthesis.
4. Nucleoside reverse transcriptase inhibitors cause toxicity of mitochondria in adipose tissue, which leads to their atrophy [116].

7.4.2 Hepatomegaly

Clinical Features
The rate of hepatomegaly varies from as low as 29% in acquired partial lipodystrophy to as high as 84% in congenital generalized lipodystrophy [117].

Pathophysiology
The etiology of hepatomegaly in lipodystrophy is indeed multifactorial; there are metabolic, genetic, and viral causes depending on the type of lipodystrophy syndrome.

1. Autoimmune hepatitis.
2. Viral-induced mitochondrial dysfunction in adipose tissue.

Table 7.3 Distribution of fat loss in lipodystrophy syndromes

Type of lipodystrophy	Distribution of adipose atrophy
Familial partial lipodystrophy (Dunnigan variety)	Loss of subcutaneous tissue fat in the extremities and trunk. Increased fat deposition in the supraclavicular region [115]
Acquired generalized lipodystrophy	A generalized progressive loss of subcutaneous tissue fat [116]
Acquired partial lipodystrophy (APL, Barraquer-Simons syndrome)	Selective loss of subcutaneous tissue fat involving the trunk, upper limbs, and head [117, 118]
Localized lipodystrophy	Medication-induced loss of subcutaneous tissue. It tends to involve sites of injection, e.g., insulin-mediated lipodystrophy [119]

Adapted from references [115–119]

Table 7.4 Mechanisms underlying other manifestations of lipodystrophy syndromes

Clinical feature	Mechanism
Acanthosis nigricans	Insulin resistance [118]
Virilization	Hyperinsulinemia-induced hyperandrogenemia [119]
Xanthomas	Hypertriglyceridemia-induced [120]
Prominent veins and muscles in the extremities	The loss of subcutaneous tissue fat makes superficial vessels more visible [120]

Adapted from Hsu [118] Tsoukas [119] and Handelsman [120]

3. Insulin resistance and hypertriglyceridemia in the setting of lipodystrophy syndromes cause nonalcoholic fatty liver disease [117].

Patients with lipodystrophy syndromes may present with acanthosis nigricans, virilization, xanthomas, or prominence of superficial venous vasculature on the extremities (Table 7.4).

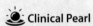 **Clinical Pearl**

Acquired Lipodystrophy Syndrome due to Immune Checkpoint Inhibitors
Immune checkpoint inhibitors are a novel class of cancer therapy used in the management of some malignancies; they are associated with untoward immune-related adverse reactions [121].

There is a single case report to date of a patient treated with nivolumab (anti-programmed cell death protein 1 monoclonal antibody) who developed an acquired form of partial lipodystrophy syndrome. The patient was severely insulin resistant and experienced progressive loss of adipose tissue in a craniocaudal direction, pathognomonic for APL [122].

APL occurred within 8 weeks of initiating nivolumab, and she was noted to have a significant loss of subcutaneous tissue fat involving the face, extremities, and gluteal regions [122].

 Questions You Might Be Asked on Clinical Rounds

What are the mechanisms responsible for the insulin resistance seen in patients with lipodystrophy syndromes?

1. *The loss of adipose tissue* reduces the storage site for free fatty acids (FFAs). Excess FFAs are alternatively stored in the liver and muscle instead. This state of lipotoxicity impairs insulin action in these peripheral tissues [119].

2. *Adiponectin*, a vital adipocytokine, *reduces hepatic glucose production* and *increases fatty acid oxidation* in the muscle. Atrophy of adipose tissue reduces the levels of this adipocytokine, which ultimately results in glucotoxicity and excess circulating FFAs. Both factors contribute to hyperinsulinemia [119].

3. Leptin, another adipocytokine, is low in the setting of adipose tissue atrophy. Leptin induces satiety through the central anorexigenic pathway – loss of leptin results in weight gain, which further exacerbates insulin resistance [119].

Which clinical features should prompt screening for lipodystrophy syndrome?

The typical distribution of subcutaneous fat loss with or without any of the following features:

1. Insulin resistance (more than 200 international units of U-100 insulin per day) [120]
2. Triglycerides ≥500 mg/dL [120]

References

1. Moosavi M, Sareshtedar A, Zarei-Ghanavati S, Zarei-Ghanavati M, Ramezanfar N. Risk factors for senile corneal arcus in patients with acute myocardial infarction. J Ophthalmic Vis Res. 2010;5:228–31.
2. Raj KM, Reddy PAS, Kumar VC. Significance of corneal arcus. J Pharm Bioallied Sci. 2015;7:S14–5.
3. Christoffersen M, Frikke-Schmidt R, Schnohr P, Jensen GB, Nordestgaard BG, Tybjærg-Hansen A. Xanthelasmata, arcus corneae, and ischaemic vascular disease and death in general population: prospective cohort study. BMJ. 2011;343:d5497.
4. Wong MYZ, Man REK, Gupta P, Lim SH, Lim B, Tham Y-C, Sabanayagam C, Wong TY, Cheng C-Y, Lamoureux EL. Is corneal arcus independently associated with incident cardiovascular disease in Asians? Am J Ophthalmol. 2017;183:99–106.
5. Christoffersen M, Tybjærg-Hansen A. Visible aging signs as risk markers for ischemic heart disease: epidemiology, pathogenesis and clinical implications. Ageing Res Rev. 2016;25:24–41.
6. Phillips CI, Tsukahara S, Gore SM. Corneal arcus: some morphology and applied pathophysiology. Jpn J Ophthalmol. 1990;34:442–9.
7. Melles G, de Sera JP, Eggink C, Cruysberg J, Binder P. Bilateral, anterior stromal ring opacity of the cornea. Br J Ophthalmol. 1998;82:522–5.
8. Zaremba J, Zaczkiewicz A, Placek W. Eruptive xanthomas. Postepy Dermatol Alergol. 2013;30:399–402.
9. Zhao C, Kong M, Cao L, Zhang Q, Fang Y, Ruan W, Dou X, Gu X, Bi Q. Multiple large xanthomas: a case report. Oncol Lett. 2016;12:4327–32.
10. Szalat R, Arnulf B, Karlin L, et al. Pathogenesis and treatment of xanthomatosis associated with monoclonal gammopathy. Blood. 2011;118:3777–84.

11. Babu R, Venkataram A, Santhosh S, Shivaswamy S. Giant tuberous xanthomas in a case of type IIA hypercholesterolemia. J Cutan Aesthet Surg. 2012;5:204–6.
12. Mastrolorenzo A, D'Errico A, Pierotti P, Vannucchi M, Giannini S, Fossi F. Pleomorphic cutaneous xanthomas disclosing homozygous familial hypercholesterolemia. World J Dermatol. 2017;6:59–65.
13. Vora RV, Kota RS, Surti NK, Singhal RR. Extensive Giant tuberous xanthomas in a 12-year-old boy. Indian Dermatol Online J. 2017;8:145–6.
14. Poonia A, Giridhara P. Xanthomas in familial hypercholesterolemia. N Engl J Med. 2017;377:e7.
15. Riche DM, East HE. Xanthomas associated with homozygous familial hypercholesterolemia. Pharmacotherapy. 2009;29:1496.
16. Sharma D, Thirkannad S. Palmar xanthoma-an indicator of a more sinister problem. Hand (N Y). 2010;5:210–2.
17. Roga G, Jithendriya M. Eruptive xanthoma: warning sign of systemic disease. Cleve Clin J Med. 2016;83:715–6.
18. Raal FJ, Santos RD. Homozygous familial hypercholesterolemia: current perspectives on diagnosis and treatment. Atherosclerosis. 2012;223:262–8.
19. Naik NS. Eruptive xanthomas. Dermatol Online J. 2001;7:11.
20. Rothschild M, Duhon G, Riaz R, Jetty V, Goldenberg N, Glueck CJ, Wang P. Pathognomonic palmar crease xanthomas of Apolipoprotein E2 homozygosity-familial Dysbetalipoproteinemia. JAMA Dermatol. 2016;152:1275–6.
21. Daroach M, Mahajan R Palmar crease xanthomas in familial hypercholesterolemia. Int J Dermatol. 58:491–2.
22. Shenoy C, Shenoy MM, Rao GK. Dyslipidemia in Dermatological Disorders. N Am J Med Sci. 2015;7:421–8.
23. Jónsson A, Sigfússon N. Letter: significance of xanthelasma palpebrarum in the normal population. Lancet. 1976;1:372.
24. Nguyen AH, Vaudreuil AM, Huerter CJ. Systematic review of laser therapy in xanthelasma palpebrarum. Int J Dermatol. 2017;56:e47–55.
25. Nair PA, Singhal R. Xanthelasma palpebrarum – a brief review. Clin Cosmet Investig Dermatol. 2017;11:1–5.
26. Laftah Z, Al-Niaimi F. Xanthelasma: an update on treatment modalities. J Cutan Aesthet Surg. 2018;11:1–6.
27. Manchanda Y, Sharma VK. Intertriginous xanthomas: a marker of homozygous type IIa hyperlipoproteinemia. Int J Dermatol. 2004;43:676–7.
28. Mete O, Kurklu E, Bilgic B, Beka H, Unur M. Flat type verruciform xanthoma of the tongue and its differential diagnosis. Dermatol Online J. 2009;15:5.
29. Griffing G. Frank's Sign. N Engl J Med. 2014;370:e15.
30. Aural Sign of Coronary-Artery Disease. New England Journal of Medicine. 1973;289:327–8.
31. Aizawa T, Shiomi H, Kitano K, Kimura T. Frank's sign: diagonal earlobe crease. Eur Heart J. 2018;39:3653.
32. Nazzal S, Hijazi B, Khalila L, Blum A. Diagonal earlobe crease (Frank's sign): a predictor of cerebral vascular events. Am J Med. 2017;130:1324.e1–5.
33. Rymarz E, Matysik-WoŸniak A, Baltaziak L, Prystupa A, Sak J, Grzybowski A. Lipemia retinalis – an unusual cause of visual acuity deterioration. Med Sci Monit. 2012;18:CS72–5.
34. Park Y-H, Lee Y-C. Lipemia Retinalis associated with secondary hyperlipidemia. N Engl J Med. 2007;357:e11.
35. Horton M, Thompson K. Lipemia retinalis preceding acute pancreatitis. Optometry- Journal of the American Optometric Association. 2011;82:475–80.
36. Hinkle JW, Relhan N, Flynn HW Jr. Lipemia Retinalis, macular edema, and vision loss in a diabetic patient with a history of type IV hypertriglyceridemia and pancreatitis. Case Rep Ophthalmol. 2018;9:425–30.
37. Zahavi A, Snir M, Kella YR. Lipemia retinalis: case report and review of the literature. Journal of American Association for Pediatric Ophthalmology and Strabismus. 2013;17:110–1.

38. Ginsberg HN. Lipoprotein physiology and its relationship to atherogenesis. Endocrinol Metab Clin N Am. 1990;19:211–28.
39. Pullinger CR, Kane JP. Lipid and lipoprotein metabolism. Reviews in Cell Biology and Molecular Medicine. 2006; https://doi.org/10.1002/3527600906.mcb.200400101.
40. Ginsberg HN. Lipoprotein physiology. Endocrinol Metab Clin N Am. 1998;27:503–19.
41. Alaupovic P. The concept of apolipoprotein-defined lipoprotein families and its clinical significance. Curr Atheroscler Rep. 2003;5:459–67.
42. Ramasamy I. Recent advances in physiological lipoprotein metabolism. Clin Chem Lab Med. 2014;52:1695–727.
43. Hussain MM. Intestinal lipid absorption and lipoprotein formation. Curr Opin Lipidol. 2014;25:200–6.
44. Iqbal J, Hussain MM. Intestinal lipid absorption. Am J Physiol Endocrinol Metab. 2009;296:E1183–94.
45. Wolska A, Dunbar RL, Freeman LA, Ueda M, Amar MJ, Sviridov DO, Remaley AT. Apolipoprotein C-II: new findings related to genetics, biochemistry, and role in triglyceride metabolism. Atherosclerosis. 2017;267:49–60.
46. Kindel T, Lee DM, Tso P. The mechanism of the formation and secretion of chylomicrons. Atheroscler Suppl. 2010;11:11–6.
47. Cohen DE, Fisher EA. Lipoprotein metabolism, dyslipidemia and nonalcoholic fatty liver disease. Semin Liver Dis. 2013;33:380–8.
48. Cooper AD. Hepatic uptake of chylomicron remnants. J Lipid Res. 1997;38:2173–92.
49. Daniels TF, Killinger KM, Michal JJ, Wright RW Jr, Jiang Z. Lipoproteins, cholesterol homeostasis and cardiac health. Int J Biol Sci. 2009;5:474–88.
50. Willnow TE. Mechanisms of hepatic chylomicron remnant clearance. Diabet Med. 1997;14(Suppl 3):S75–80.
51. Beisiegel U. Lipoprotein metabolism. Eur Heart J. 1998;19(Suppl A):A20–3.
52. Hu J, Zhang Z, Shen W-J, Azhar S. Cellular cholesterol delivery, intracellular processing and utilization for biosynthesis of steroid hormones. Nutr Metab (Lond). 2010;7:47.
53. Miller WL, Bose HS. Early steps in steroidogenesis: intracellular cholesterol trafficking. J Lipid Res. 2011;52:2111–35.
54. Bochem AE, Holleboom AG, Romijn JA, Hoekstra M, Dallinga-Thie GM, Motazacker MM, Hovingh GK, Kuivenhoven JA, Stroes ESG. High density lipoprotein as a source of cholesterol for adrenal steroidogenesis: a study in individuals with low plasma HDL-C. J Lipid Res. 2013;54:1698–704.
55. Geldenhuys WJ, Lin L, Darvesh AS, Sadana P. Emerging strategies of targeting lipoprotein lipase for metabolic and cardiovascular diseases. Drug Discov Today. 2017;22:352–65.
56. Tall AR. An overview of reverse cholesterol transport. Eur Heart J. 1998;19(Suppl a):A31–5.
57. Lin X, Racette SB, Ma L, Wallendorf M, Ostlund RE. Ezetimibe increases endogenous cholesterol excretion in humans. Arterioscler Thromb Vasc Biol. 2017;37:990–6.
58. Tall AR. Functions of cholesterol ester transfer protein and relationship to coronary artery disease risk. J Clin Lipidol. 2010;4:389–93.
59. Zhou L, Li C, Gao L, Wang A. High-density lipoprotein synthesis and metabolism (review). Mol Med Rep. 2015;12:4015–21.
60. Afonso MS, Machado RM, Lavrador MS, Quintao ECR, Moore KJ, Lottenberg AM. Molecular pathways underlying cholesterol homeostasis. Nutrients. 2018;10:760.
61. Trajkovska KT, Topuzovska S. High-density lipoprotein metabolism and reverse cholesterol transport: strategies for raising HDL cholesterol. Anatol J Cardiol. 2017;18:149–54.
62. Staels B, Fonseca VA. Bile acids and metabolic regulation. Diabetes Care. 2009;32:S237–45.
63. Pingitore P, Lepore SM, Pirazzi C, et al. Identification and characterization of two novel mutations in the LPL gene causing type I hyperlipoproteinemia. J Clin Lipidol. 2016;10:816–23.
64. Patni N, Quittner C, Garg A. Orlistat therapy for children with type 1 Hyperlipoproteinemia: a randomized clinical trial. J Clin Endocrinol Metab. 2018;103:2403–7.

65. Saint-Jore B, Varret M, Dachet C, et al. Autosomal dominant type IIa hypercholesterolemia: evaluation of the respective contributions of LDLR and APOB gene defects as well as a third major group of defects. Eur J Hum Genet. 2000;8:621–30.
66. Pejic RN. Familial hypercholesterolemia. Ochsner J. 2014;14:669–72.
67. Ellis KL, Pang J, Chan DC, Hooper AJ, Bell DA, Burnett JR, Watts GF. Familial combined hyperlipidemia and hyperlipoprotein(a) as phenotypic mimics of familial hypercholesterolemia: Frequencies, associations and predictions. J Clin Lipidol. 2016;10:1329–1337.e3.
68. Arai H, Ishibashi S, Bujo H, et al. Management of type IIb dyslipidemia. J Atheroscler Thromb. 2012;19:105–14.
69. Joerger M, Riesen WF, Thürlimann B. Bevacizumab-associated hyperlipoproteinemia type IIb in a patient with advanced invasive-ductal breast cancer. J Oncol Pharm Pract. 2011;17:292–4.
70. Hegele RA, Ban MR, Hsueh N, Kennedy BA, Cao H, Zou GY, Anand S, Yusuf S, Huff MW, Wang J. A polygenic basis for four classical Fredrickson hyperlipoproteinemia phenotypes that are characterized by hypertriglyceridemia. Hum Mol Genet. 2009;18:4189–94.
71. Brahm A, Hegele RA. Hypertriglyceridemia. Nutrients. 2013;5:981–1001.
72. Sniderman AD, de Graaf J, Thanassoulis G, Tremblay AJ, Martin SS, Couture P. The spectrum of type III hyperlipoproteinemia. J Clin Lipidol. 2018;12:1383–9.
73. Schofield JD, Liu Y, Rao-Balakrishna P, Malik RA, Soran H. Diabetes Dyslipidemia. Diabetes Ther. 2016;7:203–19.
74. Rodriguez V, Newman JD, Schwartzbard AZ. Towards more specific treatment for diabetic dyslipidemia. Curr Opin Lipidol. 2018;29:307–12.
75. Amor AJ, Perea V. Dyslipidemia in nonalcoholic fatty liver disease. Curr Opin Endocrinol Diabetes Obes. 2019;26:103.
76. Gotoda T, Shirai K, Ohta T, et al. Diagnosis and management of type I and type V hyperlipoproteinemia. J Atheroscler Thromb. 2012;19:1–12.
77. Sniderman AD, Couture P, Martin SS, DeGraaf J, Lawler PR, Cromwell WC, Wilkins JT, Thanassoulis G. Hypertriglyceridemia and cardiovascular risk: a cautionary note about metabolic confounding. J Lipid Res. 2018;59:1266–75.
78. Tenenbaum A, Klempfner R, Fisman EZ. Hypertriglyceridemia: a too long unfairly neglected major cardiovascular risk factor. Cardiovasc Diabetol. 2014;13:159.
79. Paquette M, Bernard S, Hegele RA, Baass A. Chylomicronemia: differences between familial chylomicronemia syndrome and multifactorial chylomicronemia. Atherosclerosis. 2019;283:137–42.
80. Han SH, Nicholls SJ, Sakuma I, Zhao D, Koh KK. Hypertriglyceridemia and cardiovascular diseases: revisited. Korean Circ J. 2016;46:135–44.
81. Rader DJ, de Goma EM. Approach to the patient with extremely low HDL-cholesterol. J Clin Endocrinol Metab. 2012;97:3399–407.
82. Puntoni M, Sbrana F, Bigazzi F, Sampietro T. Tangier disease: epidemiology, pathophysiology, and management. Am J Cardiovasc Drugs. 2012;12:303–11.
83. Dullaart RPF, Perton F, Sluiter WJ, de Vries R, van Tol A. Plasma lecithin: cholesterol acyltransferase activity is elevated in metabolic syndrome and is an independent marker of increased carotid artery intima media thickness. J Clin Endocrinol Metab. 2008;93:4860–6.
84. Norum KR. The function of lecithin:cholesterol acyltransferase (LCAT). Scand J Clin Lab Invest. 2017;77:235–6.
85. McIntyre N. Familial LCAT deficiency and fish-eye disease. J Inherit Metab Dis. 1988;11(Suppl 1):45–56.
86. Morales E, Alonso M, Sarmiento B, Morales M. LCAT deficiency as a cause of proteinuria and corneal opacification. BMJ Case Rep. 2018; https://doi.org/10.1136/bcr-2017-224129.
87. Kanai M, Koh S, Masuda D, Koseki M, Nishida K. Clinical features and visual function in a patient with fish-eye disease: quantitative measurements and optical coherence tomography. Am J Ophthalmol Case Rep. 2018;10:137–41.
88. Fredrickson DS, Lees RS. A system for phenotyping hyperlipoproteinemia. Circulation. 1965;31:321–7.

89. Havel RJ. Approach to the patient with hyperlipidemia. Med Clin North Am. 1982;66:319–33.
90. Khokhar AS, Seidner DL. The pathophysiology of pancreatitis. Nutr Clin Pract. 2004; 19:5–15.
91. Wasim M, Awan FR, Najam SS, Khan AR, Khan HN. Role of leptin deficiency, inefficiency, and leptin receptors in obesity. Biochem Genet. 2016;54:565–72.
92. Wabitsch M, Funcke J-B, Lennerz B, Kuhnle-Krahl U, Lahr G, Debatin K-M, Vatter P, Gierschik P, Moepps B, Fischer-Posovszky P. Biologically inactive leptin and early-onset extreme obesity. N Engl J Med. 2015;372:48–54.
93. Paz-Filho G, Mastronardi C, Delibasi T, Wong M-L, Licinio J. Congenital leptin deficiency: diagnosis and effects of leptin replacement therapy. Arq Bras Endocrinol Metabol. 2010;54:690–7.
94. Dodd G, Descherf S, Loh K, et al. Leptin and insulin act on POMC neurons to promote the browning of white fat. Cell. 2015;160:88–104.
95. Kelesidis T, Kelesidis I, Chou S, Mantzoros CS. Narrative review: the role of leptin in human physiology: emerging clinical applications. Ann Intern Med. 2010;152:93–100.
96. Saeed S, Arslan M, Froguel P. Genetics of obesity in consanguineous populations: toward precision medicine and the discovery of novel obesity genes. Obesity. 2018;26:474–84.
97. Paz-Filho G, Mastronardi CA, Licinio J. Leptin treatment: facts and expectations. Metabolism. 2015;64:146–56.
98. Paz-Filho G, Delibasi T, Erol HK, Wong M-L, Licinio J. Congenital leptin deficiency and thyroid function. Thyroid Res. 2009;2:11.
99. Krude H, Biebermann H, Luck W, Horn R, Brabant G, Grüters A. Severe early-onset obesity, adrenal insufficiency and red hair pigmentation caused by POMC mutations in humans. Nat Genet. 1998;19:155–7.
100. Ozsu E, Bahm A. Delayed diagnosis of proopiomelanocortin (POMC) deficiency with type 1 diabetes in a 9-year-old girl and her infant sibling. J Pediatr Endocrinol Metab. 2017;30:1137–40.
101. Mendiratta MS, Yang Y, Balazs AE, Willis AS, Eng CM, Karaviti LP, Potocki L. Early onset obesity and adrenal insufficiency associated with a homozygous POMC mutation. Int J Pediatr Endocrinol. 2011;2011:5.
102. Çetinkaya S, Güran T, Kurnaz E, Keskin M, Sağsak E, Savaş Erdeve S, Suntharalingham JP, Buonocore F, Achermann JC, Aycan Z. A patient with proopiomelanocortin deficiency: an increasingly important diagnosis to make. J Clin Res Pediatr Endocrinol. 2018;10:68–73.
103. Krude H, Biebermann H, Schnabel D, Tansek MZ, Theunissen P, Mullis PE, Grüters A. Obesity due to proopiomelanocortin deficiency: three new cases and treatment trials with thyroid hormone and ACTH4–10. J Clin Endocrinol Metab. 2003;88:4633–40.
104. Anisimova AS, Rubtsov PM, Akulich KA, Dmitriev SE, Frolova E, Tiulpakov A. Late diagnosis of POMC deficiency and in vitro evidence of residual translation from allele with c.-11C>a mutation. J Clin Endocrinol Metab. 2017;102:359–62.
105. Kühnen P, Clément K, Wiegand S, Blankenstein O, Gottesdiener K, Martini LL, Mai K, Blume-Peytavi U, Grüters A, Krude H. Proopiomelanocortin deficiency treated with a Melanocortin-4 receptor agonist. N Engl J Med. 2016;375:240–6.
106. Dos Videira IFS, DFL M, Magina S. Mechanisms regulating melanogenesis. An Bras Dermatol. 2013;88:76–83.
107. Pang S, Wu H, Wang Q, Cai M, Shi W, Shang J. Chronic stress suppresses the expression of cutaneous hypothalamic-pituitary-adrenocortical axis elements and melanogenesis. PLoS One. 2014;9:e98283.
108. Toda C, Santoro A, Kim JD, Diano S. POMC neurons: from birth to death. Annu Rev Physiol. 2017;79:209–36.
109. Sohn J-W. Network of hypothalamic neurons that control appetite. BMB Rep. 2015;48:229–33.
110. Zoicas F, Schöfl C. Craniopharyngioma in adults. Front Endocrin. 2012;3:46.
111. Müller HL. Craniopharyngioma. Endocr Rev. 2014;35:513–43.
112. Lustig RH. Hypothalamic obesity after Craniopharyngioma: mechanisms, diagnosis, and treatment. Front Endocrin. 2011;2:60.

113. Corvillo F, Akinci B. An overview of lipodystrophy and the role of the complement system. Mol Immunol. 2019;112:223–32.
114. Giralt M, Villarroya F, Araújo-Vilar D. Lipodystrophy. In: Huhtaniemi I, Martini L, editors. Encyclopedia of endocrine diseases. 2nd ed. Oxford: Academic Press; 2019. p. 482–95.
115. Belo SPM, Magalhães ÂC, Freitas P, Carvalho DM. Familial partial lipodystrophy, Dunnigan variety - challenges for patient care during pregnancy: a case report. BMC Res Notes. 2015;8:140.
116. Hussain I, Garg A. Lipodystrophy syndromes. Endocrinol Metab Clin N Am. 2016;45:783–97.
117. Polyzos SA, Perakakis N, Mantzoros CS. Fatty liver in lipodystrophy: a review with a focus on therapeutic perspectives of adiponectin and/or leptin replacement. Metabolism. 2019;96:66–82.
118. Hsu R-H, Lin W-D, Chao M-C, et al. Congenital generalized lipodystrophy in Taiwan. J Formos Med Assoc. 2019;118:142–7.
119. Tsoukas MA, Mantzoros CS. Chapter 37 - Lipodystrophy Syndromes. In: Jameson JL, De Groot LJ, de Kretser DM, Giudice LC, Grossman AB, Melmed S, Potts JT, Weir GC, editors. Endocrinology: adult and pediatric. 7th ed. Philadelphia: W.B. Saunders; 2016. p. 648–661.e5.
120. Handelsman Y, Oral EA, Bloomgarden ZT, et al. The clinical approach to the detection of lipodystrophy – an aace consensus statement. Endocr Pract. 2013;19:107–16.
121. Webb ES, Liu P, Baleeiro R, Lemoine NR, Yuan M, Wang Y-H. Immune checkpoint inhibitors in cancer therapy. J Biomed Res. 2018;32:317–26.
122. Falcao CK, Cabral MCS, Mota JM, et al. Acquired lipodystrophy associated with Nivolumab in a patient with advanced renal cell carcinoma. J Clin Endocrinol Metab. 2019;104:3245–8.

Eponymous Terms and Selected Historical Figures in Endocrinology

8

Learning Objectives

At the end of this chapter, you will be able to:

1. Recognize selected eponyms in the field of endocrinology, not covered in other sections of this text
2. Recall some exciting facts about the clinicians behind some notable endocrine eponyms

8.1   Eponyms Related to the Pituitary Gland

8.1.1   Wolfram Syndrome (DIDMOAD)

Clinical Features

These include diabetes insipidus, diabetes mellitus, optic nerve atrophy, and deafness (sensorineural hearing loss), hence the acronym DIDMOAD [1].

Pathophysiology

A mutation in the WFS1 gene, which encodes an endoplasmic reticulum protein, accounts for the clinical manifestations of Wolfram syndrome (WS). The endoplasmic reticulum (ER) is pivotal in mitigating the effects of cellular stress, and in the presence of WFS1 gene mutation, this protective effect is impaired, resulting in defective cellular function of nerves and pancreatic beta-cells [2].

© Springer Nature Switzerland AG 2020
A. Manni, A. Quarde, *Endocrine Pathophysiology*,
https://doi.org/10.1007/978-3-030-49872-6_8

Table 8.1 Eponyms related to the pituitary gland

Eponym	Description
Nelson's syndrome	The unregulated expansion of a pituitary tumor after bilateral adrenalectomy in patients with refractory Cushing's disease (loss of negative feedback control by adrenal-derived cortisol) [7]
Cushing's disease	Pituitary ACTH-dependent Cushing's syndrome [8]
Sheehan's syndrome	Hypopituitarism in the setting of postpartum hemorrhage [9]
Simmonds' disease	Generalized cachexia due to damage to the anterior pituitary gland [10, 11]

ACTH adrenocorticotrophic hormone
Adapted from Refs. [7–11]

8.1.2   Histiocytosis X

Clinical Features
Histiocytosis X is known by a plethora of other eponyms, including Hand-Schüller-Christian disease, Langerhans cell histiocytosis (LCH), and Letterer-Siwe disease [3]. It is a rare condition that may remain undiagnosed due to its variable presentation. Dermatologic manifestations happen to be common in subjects with LCH. The skin lesions can be suggestive of other cutaneous conditions such as eczema and seborrheic dermatitis, leading to delayed diagnosis [4]. Other physical findings include lymphadenopathy, cerebellar ataxia, tachypnea, and dehydration (central diabetes insipidus), depending on the organs involved by the disease process [5].

Pathophysiology
It is a disease of immune dysregulation involving an essential antigen-presenting cell, i.e., the dendritic cell. Despite previous controversies regarding the etiology of this condition, more recent evidence points to LCH being a neoplastic condition. Indeed, activating somatic mutations have been identified in more than 75% of patients with LCH [6]. Interestingly, LCH does not originate from cutaneous Langerhans cells, but rather derivatives of dendritic cells present in the bone marrow [3] (Table 8.1).

8.2   Eponyms Related to the Thyroid Gland

8.2.1   Pendred's Syndrome

Clinical Features
The clinical features of Pendred's syndrome include sensorineural hearing loss (SNHL), goiter, and hypothyroidism [12].

Pathophysiology

A mutation in the SLC26A4 gene, which encodes pendrin, an anion exchanger, leads to Pendred's syndrome [13]. Pendrin is a chloride-iodide cotransporter pivotal in transmembrane transport of anions in the thyroid gland, inner ear, and kidneys. It is essential in the shuttling of iodide from the thyroid follicular cell into the central colloid, a critical step required for the iodination of the thyroglobulin molecule. Pendrin is also involved in chloride and bicarbonate exchange in both the kidneys and the endolymphatic sacs. Impaired function of pendrin causes hypothyroidism, goiter, SNHL [14], and metabolic alkalosis (especially in the presence of a high bicarbonate load) [12].

 Clinical Pearl

There are a few anatomical eponyms related to the thyroid gland. These include Berry ligament (suspensory ligament of the thyroid gland) [15], Lalouette's pyramid (pyramidal lobe of the thyroid gland) [16], Zuckerkandl tubercle (a normal anatomic protrusion from the posteromedial border of the thyroid gland) [17], and thyroid artery of Neubauer (thyroidea ima artery) [18] (Table 8.2).

Table 8.2 Eponyms related to the thyroid gland

Eponym	Description
Jod-Basedow syndrome	Iodine-induced hyperthyroidism [19, 20]. "Jod" is the German word for iodine [21]. Patients with endemic goiter, euthyroid Graves' disease, and Hashimoto's thyroiditis are at risk for this condition [21, 22]
Plummer's disease	Toxic multinodular goiter [23, 24]
De Quervain's thyroiditis	Subacute granulomatous thyroiditis [25]
Hashimoto's thyroiditis	Chronic inflammatory infiltration of the thyroid gland associated with progressive fibrosis of the thyroid parenchyma [26]
Riedel's thyroiditis	A rare, benign, inflammatory condition of the thyroid with associated fibrosis of thyrocervical tissues. It can present with hypocalcemia (fibrotic infiltration of the parathyroid glands) or hypothyroidism [27]. Patients may also present with neuronal paralysis due to nerve infiltration [28]
Wolff-Chaikoff effect	A temporary reduction in thyroid hormone synthesis in the setting of an acute iodine load. The Wolff-Chaikoff effect is an adaptive response to transient changes in iodine concentration [29, 30]. There is a brief inhibition of the thyroid peroxidase enzyme after an acute iodine load. Also, impaired activity of the sodium-iodide symporter reduces further iodine uptake, an adaptation that facilitates the eventual resumption of thyroid hormone synthesis [31]
Refetoff syndrome	A syndrome of inappropriately normal or high serum TSH in the setting of thyroid hormone excess. The syndrome is also known as thyroid hormone resistance [32]
Hashitoxicosis	An initial transient hyperthyroid phase of Hashimoto's thyroiditis [33]

Adapted from Refs. [19–33]

8.3   Eponyms Related to the Adrenal Glands

8.3.1   Carney Dyad or Carney-Stratakis Syndrome

Clinical Features
Patients develop gastric gastrointestinal stromal tumors (GISTs) and paragangliomas (PGLs) [34].

Pathophysiology
An autosomal dominant mutation of the succinate dehydrogenase (SDH), an enzyme critical in the electron transport chain. SDH genes are tumor suppressor genes; as such, a loss-of-function mutation in these genes predisposes patients to tumors [35].

 Pathophysiology Pearl
The Carney triad is composed of the features of the Carney dyad (GISTs and PGLs) and pulmonary chondromas. Unlike the Carney dyad, the Carney triad occurs in the absence of a mutation in the SDH gene. A defect in the SDH gene function, however, occurs as a result of an epigenetic phenomenon characterized by hypermethylation of the SDH gene [35].

The *Carney triad* and *dyad* should be distinguished from the classic *Carney complex* (see Table 8.3).

Table 8.3   Eponyms related to the adrenal glands

Eponym	Description
Addison's disease	Primary adrenal insufficiency characterized by glucocorticoid, androgen, and mineralocorticoid deficiency [39, 40]
Conn's syndrome	Primary hyperaldosteronism with adrenal adenoma(s) [41]
Schmidt's syndrome	Addison's disease associated with autoimmune thyroid disease in patients with polyglandular autoimmune syndrome type 2 [42]
Carpenter's syndrome	Schmidt's syndrome with associated type 1 diabetes mellitus in patients with polyglandular autoimmune syndrome type 2 [42, 43]
Cushing's syndrome	Hypercortisolemia due to a cortisol secreting tumor, pituitary, or ectopic source of excess adrenocorticotropic hormone (ACTH) production or exposure to supraphysiologic levels of exogenous glucocorticoids [44, 45]
Addisonian anemia	Pernicious anemia in the setting of Addison's disease [46]
Carney complex	A mutation in the gene encoding the type 1 alpha subunit of protein kinase A is implicated in the Carney complex. Clinical features include functional pituitary tumors, cardiac myxomas, café-au-lait macules, and ACTH-independent hypercortisolemia (PPNAD) [47]

PPNAD primary pigmented nodular adrenocortical disease
Adapted from Refs. [39–47]

8.3.2 Allgrove Syndrome

Clinical Features
Allgrove or triple A syndrome is composed of a triad of achalasia, alacrimia (absence of tears), and adrenal insufficiency [36]. Adrenal insufficiency contributes significantly to the morbidity and mortality observed in patients with Allgrove syndrome [37].

Pathophysiology
Triple A syndrome occurs as a result of a mutation in the *AAAS* gene, which encodes a protein called ALADIN. ALADIN is critical in maintaining the integrity of cellular membranes [38], control of steroidogenesis, and redox reactions in the adrenal gland [37].

8.4 Eponyms Related to the Pancreas

8.4.1 Kussmaul's Breathing (Diabetic Ketoacidosis)

Clinical Features
Patients with severe metabolic acidosis as might occur in diabetic ketoacidosis develop a terminal, deep, and rapid respiratory pattern called Kussmaul's respiration. It heralds an impending state of respiratory failure requiring assisted ventilation [48]. A characteristic fruity odor due to acetone, often described as similar to the smell of nail polish remover, can be appreciated during the physical examination [49].

Pathophysiology
Metabolic acidosis triggers a compensatory increase in the respiratory rate in order to reduce dissolved carbon dioxide and thus maintain serum pH. An initial phase of tachypnea progresses through hyperpnea (increased tidal volume) and culminates into the preterminal respiratory pattern of Kussmaul's respiration [48].

Kussmaul's respiration, a compensatory response to metabolic acidosis, increases intra-alveolar pressures and may predispose patients to alveolar rupture and pneumomediastinum (Hamman's syndrome) [50].

8.4.2 Somogyi Effect

Clinical Features
The Somogyi effect has classically been described as rebound early-morning hyperglycemia in the setting of significant fasting, overnight hypoglycemia. This colorful eponym in diabetology was first reported by Michael Somogyi in 1959 [51].

Table 8.4 Eponyms related to the pancreas

Eponym	Description
Wermer's syndrome	Multiple endocrine neoplasia type 1 (pancreatic tumors, parathyroid tumors, pituitary tumors, adrenal cortical tumors, and schwannomas) [53]
Whipple's triad	A triad of hypoglycemic symptoms, biochemically confirmed hypoglycemia, and reversal of hypoglycemic symptomatology after correction of hypoglycemia [54]
Zollinger-Ellison syndrome	Hypergastrinemia in the setting of a pancreatic gastrin-secreting neuroendocrine tumor [55, 56]. Most gastrinomas occur in the *gastrinoma triangle*, which is an imaginary triangle drawn through the pancreatic head, porta hepatis, and the transition point between the second and third parts of the duodenum [55]
Verner-Morrison syndrome	Syndrome of chronic watery diarrhea, hypokalemia, and achlorhydria (WDHA syndrome) occurs in patients with vasoactive intestinal peptide-secreting pancreatic neuroendocrine tumors [57]

Adapted from Refs. [53–57]

Pathophysiology
The long-held belief has been that a period of hypoglycemia during an overnight fast triggers a counterregulatory hormonal response, which results in fasting hyperglycemia in the morning [52]. In a prospective study involving 262 subjects, the investigators used continuous glucose monitoring to assess trends in glycemic control among patients on a basal-bolus regimen. In subjects who developed nocturnal hypoglycemia, fasting hyperglycemia in the morning did not occur, discounting the Somogyi effect as a cause of fasting hyperglycemia [51] (Table 8.4).

8.5 Eponyms Related to the Parathyroid Glands and Bone Metabolism

8.5.1 Albers-Schönberg Disease

Clinical Features
Autosomal dominant osteopetrosis type 2 (ADO2) is also known as Albers-Schönberg disease. The clinical features of this disease include nontraumatic fractures, cranial nerve palsies, and osteoarthritis [58].

Pathophysiology
A series of genetic mutations leading to defective bone resorption have been implicated in the etiopathogenesis of osteopetrosis [58, 59]. Expansion of cortical bone results in craniofacial changes (including macrocephaly) and compressive neuropathies. Bone mineral density is significantly high due to impaired osteoclastic activity, although this is paradoxically associated with increased fragility fractures [60].

Table 8.5 Eponyms related to the parathyroid glands and bone metabolism

Eponym	Description
Albright's hereditary osteodystrophy	Shortened fourth metacarpals or metatarsals in patients with pseudohypoparathyroidism or pseudopseudohypoparathyroidism [62]
Von Recklinghausen's disease of bone	Osteitis fibrosa cystica with the formation of peculiar brown tumors [63]
Albright's anemia	Association of primary hyperparathyroidism with anemia [64, 65]
DiGeorge syndrome	Hypoparathyroidism, congenital heart disease, and a poorly developed thymus [66]
Sipple's syndrome	Multiple endocrine neoplasia type 2A (medullary thyroid cancer, pheochromocytomas, and parathyroid hyperplasia or adenomas) [53]

Adapted from Refs. [53, 62–66]

8.5.2   McCune-Albright Syndrome

Clinical Features
McCune-Albright syndrome is characterized by fibrous dysplasia of bone, sexual precocity, and characteristic macular lesions called "café-au-lait" skin pigmentation [61].

Pathophysiology
Mutation in the GNAS gene, which encodes the alpha subunit of the stimulatory G-protein, is implicated in this syndrome. The mutation results in *constitutive activation* (activation in the absence of hormonal stimulation) of this G-protein, which fuels most of the downstream effects of several hormones. Patients can present hyperthyroidism, precocious puberty, fibrous dysplasia, growth hormone excess, and Cushing's syndrome [61] (Table 8.5).

8.6   Miscellaneous Eponyms

Additional eponyms in endocrinology are briefly outlined in Table 8.6.

8.7   A Brief Account of Selected Historical Figures in Endocrinology

8.7.1   Harvey Cushing (1869–1939)

Harvey Cushing, a graduate of Harvard Medical School (1891–1896). A neurosurgeon by training who became internationally recognized in the early 1900s. He made significant contributions to the field of neurosurgery and is known as the father of modern neurosurgery. He, however, holds a special place in clinical endocrinology due to his description of "pituitary basophilia" or Cushing's disease, a clinical syndrome eponymously named after him [74].

Table 8.6 Additional miscellaneous eponyms

Eponym	Description
Stein-Leventhal syndrome	Polycystic ovarian syndrome [67]

Von Hippel-Lindau syndrome	*Germline mutation in the VHL tumor suppressor gene*
	  Pheochromocytomas
	  Renal cell carcinomas
	  Central nervous system hemangioblastomas
	  Pancreatic cysts [68]

Von Recklinghausen's disease	*Neurofibromatosis type 1. Mutation of NF-1 tumor suppressor gene*
	  Café-au-lait skin pigmentation
	  Axillary (Crowe's sign) and inguinal freckles
	  Neurofibromas
	  Pheochromocytomas
	  Eye manifestations (optic gliomas and pigmented hamartomas involving the iris) [69]

Mayer-Rokitansky-Kuster-Hauser (MRKH) syndrome	Agenesis of the Mullerian duct. The genetic basis is still under investigation. Congenital Mullerian abnormalities ranging from minor anomalies to total aplasia of Mullerian derivatives [70]
Burger-Grutz syndrome	Lipoprotein lipase (LPL) deficiency due to a genetic mutation in the LPL gene. Classified as Fredrickson type 1 hyperlipidemia Xanthomas, lipemia retinalis, hepatosplenomegaly, and pancreatitis [71]
Montgomery's syndrome	It is also referred to as *xanthoma disseminatum (XD)*. Generalized xanthomas involving the skin and mucous membranes in the absence of hyperlipidemia [72] and may be associated with diabetes insipidus [73]

Adapted from Refs. [67–73]

 Medical Trivia

1. Harvey Cushing's mentor was William Osler, a name known by many a medical trainee. They formed a professional and personal relationship during their time together at Johns Hopkins Hospital in Maryland. He wrote a two-volume biography of Osler in 1925.
2. The anesthesia record, which details a patient's vital signs during surgery, is credited to him.
3. Other non-endocrine eponyms bearing his name include Cushing's ulcers and Cushing's reflex [75].

8.7.2   Hakaru Hashimoto (1881–1934)

Hakaru Hashimoto, a graduate of Fukuoka Medical College (1903–1907). He reported a case series of a previously unknown form of thyroid disease. Four female patients aged 40 years and older underwent partial thyroidectomy and were found to have the characteristic histological findings of chronic lymphocytic thyroiditis.

Hashimoto used the term *struma lymphomatosa* to describe the unique chronic inflammation of the thyroid gland [76]. Chronic lymphocytic thyroiditis is eponymously named "Hashimoto's thyroiditis" [77].

Hashimoto compared his findings with those reported in Riedel's thyroiditis. Patients with struma lymphomatosa, however, had less fibrosis noted on histology. Also, the thyroid gland of his subjects on clinical examination did not have the hard consistency of Riedel's thyroiditis, which made it a distinct clinical entity [78].

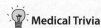 **Medical Trivia**

1. Hashimoto's discovery was mostly unrecognized for decades. His findings were again reported by another clinician who seemingly was unaware of Hashimoto's original paper from 1912. He was eventually recognized at an international thyroid conference in 1938 [78].
2. His paper on struma lymphomatosa was initially published in the German language [79].

8.7.3   Thomas Addison (1793–1860)

Thomas Addison graduated from the University of Edinburgh Medical School in 1815. *Addison's anemia* was first reported in the *London Medical Gazette* in 1849 as "Anaemia – disease of the suprarenal capsules in which the disease is not distinctly separated from a new form of anemia." Trousseau (1801–1867) was the first to use the eponym "Addison's disease" [80].

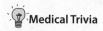 **Medical Trivia**

1. Pernicious anemia is eponymously called *Addison's anemia* [81].
2. The classical description of *vitiligo* is credited to Addison [81].

8.7.4   Fuller Albright (1900–1969)

Fuller Albright enrolled at Harvard Medical School in 1920. His research findings have been influential in our understanding of calcium and bone metabolism. He shares the eponymous term, *McCune-Albright syndrome,* with Donovan McCune.

He also made significant contributions to our understanding of osteoporosis, hyperparathyroidism, and Cushing's disease [82].

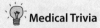Medical Trivia

1. Albright had an initial desire to become an orthopedic surgeon but had to shelve those dreams because he did not have the dexterity required in this surgical subdiscipline. He was fascinated by calcium metabolism and subsequently turned his interests to the field of endocrinology [82].

   He investigated the role of estrogen in bone metabolism and postulated that estrogens stimulate osteoblast function and thus improve bone health [82]. Albright developed Parkinson's disease when he was 36 years of age and unfortunately, suffered an intracranial hemorrhage during a pallidotomy, a novel procedure at the time for Parkinson's disease [82].

8.7.5   Jerome W. Conn (1907–1994)

Jerome W. Conn, a graduate of the University of Michigan Medical School (1929–1932). He made a lasting contribution to our understanding of the renin-angiotensin-aldosterone axis [83]. Primary hyperaldosteronism due to a unilateral aldosterone-secreting tumor is widely reported as *Conn's syndrome* [84].

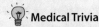Medical Trivia

1. Conn had an interest in diabetes pathophysiology, and his publications have provided insights into our understanding of insulin-resistant states [85].
2. Jerome Conn completed a year of training in general surgery, but redirected his interests to internal medicine and, subsequently, endocrinology [85].

8.7.6   Frederick Banting (1891–1941)

Frederick Banting completed his medical education at the University of Toronto in 1916. He is known for the discovery of insulin, an honor he graciously shared with a junior colleague, Charles H. Best [86].

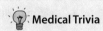Medical Trivia

Banting and J.R.R Macleod were awarded the Nobel Prize in Medicine and Physiology in 1923 [87].

8.7.7   Robert Graves (1797–1853)

Robert Graves completed his medical education at the University of Dublin in 1818. He described exophthalmic goiter but was arguably not the first to describe this malady. von Basedow and others documented the clinical features of diffuse toxic goiter before Robert Graves. Graves' disease is also referred to as Basedow's disease in some medical circles [88].

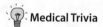 **Medical Trivia**

1. He described the "pinpoint" pupillary findings in patients with a pontine hemorrhage.
2. Graves advocated for discontinuation of the practice of phlebotomy as a means of treating pyrexia.
3. He proposed the concept of timing of peripheral pulses [88].

8.7.8   Edward Kendall (1888–1972)

Edward Kendall completed his BSc, MSc and Ph.D. degrees at Columbia University, New York City. He shared the 1950 Nobel Prize for Medicine and Physiology with Philip Hench (1896–1965), for the discovery of cortisone [89].

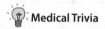 **Medical Trivia**

1. Kendall crystallized thyroxine in 1914, during his time at Mayo Clinic (Rochester, Minnesota).
2. He isolated at least 28 adrenocortical hormones, including cortisone, a hormone he initially designated as "compound E" [89].

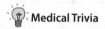 **Clinical Pearl**

Occam's Razor
   A principle in medicine that posits that a single unifying diagnosis should be considered as an explanation for multiple presenting symptoms [90]
   Hickam's Dictum
   A principle in medicine which reminds clinicians of the importance of recognizing that two or more distinct diagnoses can co-exist in the same patient [91]. Humorously, this is sometimes referred to as the dictum of fleas and lice, which states, "A diagnosis of fleas does not exclude a diagnosis of lice in the same patient" [92].

References

1. Barrett TG, Bundey SE. Wolfram (DIDMOAD) syndrome. J Med Genet. 1997;34:838–41.
2. Urano F. Wolfram syndrome: diagnosis, management, and treatment. Curr Diab Rep. 2016;16:6.
3. Kobayashi M, Tojo A. Langerhans cell histiocytosis in adults: advances in pathophysiology and treatment. Cancer Sci. 2018;109:3707–13.
4. Simko SJ, Garmezy B, Abhyankar H, et al. Differentiating skin-limited and multisystem Langerhans cell histiocytosis. J Pediatr. 2014;165:990–6.
5. Haupt R, Minkov M, Astigarraga I, et al. Langerhans cell histiocytosis (LCH): guidelines for diagnosis, clinical work-up, and treatment for patients till the age of 18 years. Pediatr Blood Cancer. 2013;60:175–84.
6. Jezierska M, Stefanowicz J, Romanowicz G, Kosiak W, Lange M. Langerhans cell histiocytosis in children – a disease with many faces. Recent advances in pathogenesis, diagnostic examinations and treatment. Postepy Dermatol Alergol. 2018;35:6–17.
7. Barber TM, Adams E, JAH W. Nelson syndrome: definition and management. Handb Clin Neurol. 2014;124:327–37.
8. Castinetti F, Morange I, Conte-Devolx B, Brue T. Cushing's disease. Orphanet J Rare Dis. 2012;7:41.
9. Kilicli F, Dokmetas HS, Acibucu F. Sheehan's syndrome. Gynecol Endocrinol. 2013;29:292–5.
10. Rosenberg B, Rosenthal J, Beck GJ. Simmonds' disease; case reports. Am J Med. 1948;5:462–9.
11. Beare JM. Simmonds' disease. Ulster Med J. 1947;16:66–42.10.
12. Wémeau J-L, Kopp P. Pendred syndrome. Best Pract Res Clin Endocrinol Metab. 2017;31:213–24.
13. Bizhanova A, Kopp P. Genetics and phenomics of Pendred syndrome. Mol Cell Endocrinol. 2010;322:83–90.
14. Smith N, U-King-Im J-M, Karalliedde J. Delayed diagnosis of Pendred syndrome. BMJ Case Rep. 2016;2016:bcr2016215271.
15. Rajabian A, Walsh M, Quraishi NA. Berry's ligament and the inferior thyroid artery as reliable anatomical landmarks for the recurrent laryngeal nerve (RLN): a fresh-cadaveric study of the cervical spine. The RLN relevant to spine. Spine J. 2017;17:S33–9.
16. Akudu LS, Ukoha UU, Ekezie J, Ukoha CC. Ultrasonographic study of the incidence of pyramidal lobe and agenesis of the thyroid isthmus in Nnewi population. J Ultrason. 2018;18:290–5.
17. Won H-J, Won H-S, Kwak D-S, Jang J, Jung S-L, Kim I-B. Zuckerkandl tubercle of the thyroid gland: correlations between findings of anatomic dissections and CT imaging. AJNR Am J Neuroradiol. 2017;38:1416–20.
18. Kamparoudi P, Paliouras D, Gogakos AS, et al. Percutaneous tracheostomy—beware of the thyroidea-ima artery. Ann Transl Med. 2016;4:449.
19. Dave A, Ludlow J, Malaty J. Thyrotoxicosis: an under-recognised aetiology. BMJ Case Rep. 2015;2015:bcr2014208119.
20. De Leo S, Braverman LE. Iodine-induced thyroid dysfunction. In: Luster M, Duntas LH, Wartofsky L, editors. The thyroid and its diseases: a comprehensive guide for the clinician. Cham: Springer International Publishing; 2019. p. 435–52.
21. Chung HR. Iodine and thyroid function. Ann Pediatr Endocrinol Metab. 2014;19:8–12.
22. Dunne P, Kaimal N, MacDonald J, Syed AA. Iodinated contrast–induced thyrotoxicosis. CMAJ. 2013;185:144–7.
23. Porterfield JR, Thompson GB, Farley DR, Grant CS, Richards ML. Evidence-based management of toxic multinodular goiter (Plummer's disease). World J Surg. 2008;32:1278–84.
24. Ngalob QG, Isip-Tan IT. Thyroid cancer in Plummer's disease. BMJ Case Rep. 2013;2013:bcr2013008909.
25. Ranganath R, Shaha MA, Xu B, Migliacci J, Ghossein R, Shaha AR. de Quervain's thyroiditis: a review of experience with surgery. Am J Otolaryngol. 2016;37:534–7.

26. Zaletel K, Gaberšček S. Hashimoto's thyroiditis: from genes to the disease. Curr Genomics. 2011;12:576–88.
27. Hennessey JV. Clinical review: Riedel's thyroiditis: a clinical review. J Clin Endocrinol Metab. 2011;96:3031–41.
28. Ng SA, Corcuera-Solano I, Gurudutt VV, Som PM. A rare case of Reidel thyroiditis with associated vocal cord paralysis: CT and MR imaging features. AJNR Am J Neuroradiol. 2011;32:E201–2.
29. Leung AM, Braverman LE. Consequences of excess iodine. Nat Rev Endocrinol. 2014;10:136–42.
30. Okamura K, Sato K, Fujikawa M, Bandai S, Ikenoue H, Kitazono T. Remission after potassium iodide therapy in patients with graves' hyperthyroidism exhibiting thionamide-associated side effects. J Clin Endocrinol Metab. 2014;99:3995–4002.
31. Pramyothin P, Leung AM, Pearce EN, Malabanan AO, Braverman LE. Clinical problem-solving. A hidden solution. N Engl J Med. 2011;365:2123–7.
32. Alberto G, Novi RF, Scalabrino E, Trombetta A, Seardo MA, Maurino M, Brossa C. Atrial fibrillation and mitral prolapse in a subject affected by Refetoff syndrome. Minerva Cardioangiol. 2002;50:157–60.
33. Nabhan ZM, Kreher NC, Eugster EA. Hashitoxicosis in children: clinical features and natural history. J Pediatr. 2005;146:533–6.
34. Szarek E, Ball ER, Imperiale A, et al. Carney Triad, SDH-deficient tumors, and Sdhb+/− mice share abnormal mitochondria. Endocr Relat Cancer. 2015;22:345–52.
35. Settas N, Faucz FR, Stratakis CA. Succinate dehydrogenase (SDH) deficiency, carney triad and the epigenome. Mol Cell Endocrinol. 2018;469:107–11.
36. de Freitas MRG, Orsini M, et al. Allgrove syndrome and motor neuron disease. Neurol Int. 2018;10(2):7436. https://doi.org/10.4081/ni.2018.7436.
37. Brown B, Agdere L, Muntean C, David K. Alacrima as a harbinger of adrenal insufficiency in a child with Allgrove (AAA) syndrome. Am J Case Rep. 2016;17:703–6.
38. Li W, Gong C, Qi Z, Wu D, Cao B. Identification of AAAS gene mutation in Allgrove syndrome: a report of three cases. Exp Ther Med. 2015;10:1277–82.
39. Bornstein SR, Allolio B, Arlt W, et al. Diagnosis and treatment of primary adrenal insufficiency: an endocrine society clinical practice guideline. J Clin Endocrinol Metab. 2016;101:364–89.
40. Burton C, Cottrell E, Edwards J. Addison's disease: identification and management in primary care. Br J Gen Pract. 2015;65:488–90.
41. Funder JW, Carey RM, Mantero F, Murad MH, Reincke M, Shibata H, Stowasser M, Young WF. The management of primary aldosteronism: case detection, diagnosis, and treatment: an endocrine society clinical practice guideline. J Clin Endocrinol Metab. 2016;101:1889–916.
42. Dittmar M, Kahaly GJ. Polyglandular autoimmune syndromes: immunogenetics and long-term follow-up. J Clin Endocrinol Metab. 2003;88:2983–92.
43. Carpenter CC, Solomon N, Silverberg SG, Bledsoe T, Northcutt RC, Klinenberg JR, Bennett IL, Harvey AM. Schmidt's syndrome (thyroid and adrenal insufficiency). A review of the literature and a report of fifteen new cases including ten instances of coexistent diabetes mellitus. Medicine (Baltimore). 1964;43:153–80.
44. Lacroix A, Feelders RA, Stratakis CA, Nieman LK. Cushing's syndrome. Lancet. 2015;386:913–27.
45. Pappachan JM, Hariman C, Edavalath M, Waldron J, Hanna FW. Cushing's syndrome: a practical approach to diagnosis and differential diagnoses. J Clin Pathol. 2017;70:350–9.
46. Kra SJ, Barile AW. Addison's disease and Addisonian Anemia: a case report. Arch Intern Med. 1964;114:258–62.
47. Correa R, Salpea P, Stratakis CA. Carney complex: an update. Eur J Endocrinol. 2015;173:M85–97.
48. Gallo de Moraes A, Surani S. Effects of diabetic ketoacidosis in the respiratory system. World J Diabetes. 2019;10:16–22.
49. Seth P, Kaur H, Kaur M. Clinical profile of diabetic ketoacidosis: a prospective study in a tertiary care hospital. J Clin Diagn Res. 2015;9:OC01–4.

50. Pain AR, Pomroy J, Benjamin A. Hamman's syndrome in diabetic ketoacidosis. Endocrinol Diabetes Metab Case Rep. 2017;1(1):1–4. https://doi.org/10.1530/EDM-17-0135.
51. Høi-Hansen T, Pedersen-Bjergaard U, Thorsteinsson B. The Somogyi phenomenon revisited using continuous glucose monitoring in daily life. Diabetologia. 2005;48:2437–8.
52. Rybicka M, Krysiak R, Okopień B. The dawn phenomenon and the Somogyi effect - two phenomena of morning hyperglycaemia. Endokrynol Pol. 2011;62:276–84.
53. Vandersteen PR, Scheithauer BW. Glucagonoma syndrome. J Am Acad Dermatol. 1985;12:1032–9.
54. Kong M-F, Lawden M, Dennison A. Altered mental state and the Whipple triad. BMJ Case Rep. 2010; https://doi.org/10.1136/bcr.08.2009.2158.
55. Epelboym I, Mazeh H. Zollinger-Ellison syndrome: classical considerations and current controversies. Oncologist. 2014;19:44–50.
56. Singh Ospina N, Donegan D, Rodriguez-Gutierrez R, Al-Hilli Z, Young WF. Assessing for multiple endocrine neoplasia type 1 in patients evaluated for Zollinger-Ellison syndrome-clues to a safer diagnostic process. Am J Med. 2017;130:603–5.
57. Belei OA, Heredea ER, Boeriu E, Marcovici TM, Cerbu S, Mărginean O, Iacob ER, Iacob D, Motoc AGM, Boia ES. Verner-Morrison syndrome. Literature review. Romanian J Morphol Embryol. 2017;58:371–6.
58. Cleiren E, Bénichou O, Van Hul E, et al. Albers-Schönberg disease (autosomal dominant osteopetrosis, type II) results from mutations in the ClCN7 chloride channel gene. Hum Mol Genet. 2001;10:2861–7.
59. Sobacchi C, Schulz A, Coxon FP, Villa A, Helfrich MH. Osteopetrosis: genetics, treatment and new insights into osteoclast function. Nat Rev Endocrinol. 2013;9:522–36.
60. Stark Z, Savarirayan R. Osteopetrosis. Orphanet J Rare Dis. 2009;4:5.
61. Salpea P, Stratakis CA. Carney complex and McCune Albright syndrome: an overview of clinical manifestations and human molecular genetics. Mol Cell Endocrinol. 2014;386:85–91.
62. Rolla AR, Rodriguez-Gutierrez R. Albright's hereditary osteodystrophy. N Engl J Med. 2012;367:2527.
63. Vaishya R, Agarwal AK, Singh H, Vijay V. Multiple "Brown tumors" masquerading as metastatic bone disease. Cureus. 2015;7:e431.
64. Mallette LE. Anemia in hypercalcemic hyperparathyroidism: renewed interest in an old observation. Arch Intern Med. 1977;137:572–3.
65. Baskaran LNGM, Greco PJ, Kaelber DC. Case report medical eponyms. Appl Clin Inform. 2012;3:349–55.
66. McDonald-McGinn DM, Sullivan KE, Marino B, et al. 22q11.2 deletion syndrome. Nat Rev Dis Primers. 2015;1:15071.
67. Kurzrock R, Cohen PR. Polycystic ovary syndrome in men: Stein-Leventhal syndrome revisited. Med Hypotheses. 2007;68:480–3.
68. Maher ER, Neumann HP, Richard S. von Hippel–Lindau disease: a clinical and scientific review. Eur J Hum Genet. 2011;19:617–23.
69. Ghalayani P, Saberi Z, Sardari F. Neurofibromatosis type I (von Recklinghausen's disease): a family case report and literature review. Dent Res J (Isfahan). 2012;9:483–8.
70. Fontana L, Gentilin B, Fedele L, Gervasini C, Miozzo M. Genetics of Mayer-Rokitansky-Küster-Hauser (MRKH) syndrome. Clin Genet. 2017;91:233–46.
71. Viljoen A, Wierzbicki AS. Diagnosis and treatment of severe hypertriglyceridemia. Expert Rev Cardiovasc Ther. 2012;10:505–14.
72. Banerjee M, Sharma P, Gaur N, Takkar B. Infiltrative chiasmatopathy in xanthoma disseminatum: a rare entity. BMJ Case Rep. 2018;11:e227207.
73. Beurey J, Lamaze B, Weber M, Delrous JL, Kremer B, Chaulieu Y. Xanthoma disseminatum (Montgomery's syndrome) (author's transl). Ann Dermatol Venereol. 1979;106:353–9.
74. Perrins RJ. Harvey cushing: a life in surgery. Soc Hist Med. 2006;19:576–8.
75. Loriaux DL. Harvey Williams Cushing (1869–1939). In: A biographical history of endocrinology. D.L. Loriaux (Ed.). Wiley; 2016. p. 202–6. https://doi.org/10.1002/9781119205791.ch48.

76. Loriaux DL. Hakaru Hashimoto (1881–1934). In: A biographical history of endocrinology. D.L. Loriaux (Ed.). Wiley; 2016. p. 269–73. https://doi.org/10.1002/9781119205791.ch61.
77. Graham A, McCullagh EP. Atrophy and fibrosis associated with lymphoid tissue in the thyroid: struma lymphomatosa (Hashimoto). Arch Surg. 1931;22:548–67.
78. Sawin CT. Hakaru Hashimoto (1881–1934) and his disease. Endocrinologist. 2001;11:73–6.
79. Volpé R. The life of Dr. Hakaru Hashimoto. Autoimmunity. 1989;3:243–5.
80. Pearce JMS. Thomas Addison (1793-1860). J R Soc Med. 2004;97:297–300.
81. Jay V. Thomas addison. Arch Pathol Lab Med. 1999;123:190.
82. Manring MM, Calhoun JH. Biographical sketch: Fuller Albright, MD 1900–1969. Clin Orthop Relat Res. 2011;469:2092–5.
83. Fajans SS. Jerome W. Conn, 1907–1994. Ann Intern Med. 1994;121:901.
84. Christakis I, Livesey JA, Sadler GP, Mihai R. Laparoscopic Adrenalectomy for Conn's syndrome is beneficial to patients and is cost effective in England. J Investig Surg. 2018;31:300–6.
85. Loriaux D. Jerome W. Conn (1907–1994). Endocrinologist. 2008;18:159–60.
86. Tan SY, Merchant J. Frederick Banting (1891–1941): discoverer of insulin. Singap Med J. 2017;58:2–3.
87. Bliss M. "Texts and documents": Banting's, Best's, and Collip's accounts of the discovery of insulin. Bull History Med. 1982;56:554.
88. Jay V. Dr Robert James Graves. Arch Pathol Lab Med. 1999;123:284.
89. Shampo MA, Kyle RA. Edward C. Kendall—Nobel Laureate. Mayo Clin Proc. 2001;76:1188.
90. Freixa M, Simões AF, Rodrigues JB, Úria S, da Silva GN. Occam's razor versus Hickam's dictum: two very rare tumours in one single patient. Oxf Med Case Rep. 2019;2019(5):omz029. https://doi.org/10.1093/omcr/omz029.
91. Wilkinson ST, Grunwald MR, Paik JJ, Ostrow LW, Gelber AC. Hickam's dictum and the rare convergence of antisynthetase syndrome and hemoglobin SC disease. QJM. 2015;108:735–7.
92. Neiman ES, Farheen A, Gadallah N, Steineke T, Parsells P, Kizelnik ZA, Rosenberg M. An unusual presentation of Creutzfeldt-Jakob disease and an example of how Hickam's dictum and Ockham's razor can both be right. Neurodiagn J. 2017;57:234–9.

Appendix

Appendix 1: Selected Genetic Mutations and Their Corresponding Endocrine States

Table A.1 Pituitary gland

Gene(s)	Endocrine condition
AIP	Familial isolated pituitary adenoma (FIPA) syndrome
KAL1, FGFR1	Kallmann syndrome
PROP1, POUF1F1	Combined pituitary hormone deficiency
Menin	Multiple endocrine neoplasia type 1
PRKAR1A	Carney complex
GnRH-1, KISS 1	Normosmic idiopathic hypogonadotropic hypogonadism (IHH)
DAX1	Normosmic IHH and adrenal insufficiency
LEP	Normosmic IHH and obesity

Table A.2 Thyroid gland

Gene(s)	Endocrine condition
SCN4A	Hypokalemic periodic paralysis
SLC26A4	Pendred's syndrome
PAX8, TSHR	Congenital hypothyroidism
THRB, THRA	Thyroid hormone resistance

Table A.3 Adrenal gland

Gene(s)	Endocrine condition
ALADIN	Triple A syndrome (primary adrenal insufficiency, alacrima, and achalasia)
RET	Multiple endocrine neoplasia types 2A and 2B
TSC1, TSC2	Tuberous sclerosis complex
VHL	Von Hippel-Lindau syndrome
ABCD1	X-linked adrenoleukodystrophy
MC2R	Familial glucocorticoid deficiency
SDHx	Hereditary pheochromocytoma-paraganglioma syndromes
TP53	Adrenocortical carcinoma
KCNJ5	Familial hyperaldosteronism

SDHx refers to SDHA, SDHB, SDHB, and SDHAF2

© Springer Nature Switzerland AG 2020
A. Manni, A. Quarde, *Endocrine Pathophysiology*,
https://doi.org/10.1007/978-3-030-49872-6

Table A.4 Pancreatic gland

Gene(s)	Endocrine condition
GCK	Monogenic diabetes (uncomplicated course)
HNF1A	Monogenic diabetes (sulfonylurea responsive)
WFS1	Wolfram syndrome (DIDMOAD)
KCNJ11	Neonatal diabetes
ABCC8, KCNJ11	Congenital hyperinsulinism

Table A.5 Parathyroid gland, calcium, and bone metabolism

Gene(s)	Endocrine condition
CASR	Familial hypocalciuric hypercalcemia
ELN	Williams-Beuren syndrome
AIRE	Autoimmune polyglandular syndrome type 1
COL1A1, COL1A2	Osteogenesis imperfecta
GCM2, PTH	Familial isolated hypoparathyroidism
22q11.2	DiGeorge syndrome
PHEX	Hereditary hypophosphatemic rickets

Table A.6 Lipids and obesity

Gene(s)	Endocrine condition
CETP	CETP deficiency
ABCA1	Tangier disease
LEP	Congenital leptin deficiency
Apo C-II	Hypertriglyceridemia-related disorders
LPL	Hypertriglyceridemia-related disorders
LDL-R, PCSK-9	Familial hypercholesterolemia
LCAT	Familial LCAT deficiency
MTP	Abetalipoproteinemia
Apo E	Dysbetalipoproteinemia
ABCG5	Sitosterolemia

Appendix 2: Examination of the Thyroid Gland, an Endocrine Approach

Illustration of the optimal position of the palms and use of the second, third, and fourth digits in palpating the thyroid gland in the low anterior neck

Our approach involves sequentially inspecting, palpating, percussing (where relevant), and auscultating the thyroid.

Inspection of the Thyroid Gland

- A visible anterior neck mass, which is mobile on deglutition, implies an enlarged gland. Offer the patient a glass of water to drink. The normal thyroid gland cannot be visualized on inspection.
- Positive *Pemberton's sign* is suggestive of significant retrosternal extension of a goiter.

Fig. A.1 Examination of
the thyroid gland

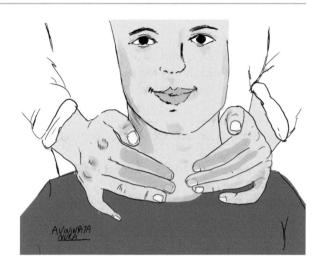

Palpation

- Optimal positioning of the neck will facilitate palpation of the gland. The patient's neck should be in a relaxed position, which prevents extensive nuchal extension or flexion. The sternocleidomastoid muscle should not be under tension, and there should be adequate room between the chin and the sternum to allow proper positioning of the hands.
- Sequentially palpate each thyroid lobe and isthmus. Occasionally there might be an accessory extension of the isthmus – the pyramidal lobe. Check for the consistency of the gland. Avoid deep palpation if the gland is tender, as might occur in De Quervain's thyroiditis. The normal thyroid has a mild firm consistency. The overlying skin is usually freely mobile over it. If the gland is attached to the overlying skin, it might be suggestive of either a malignancy or Riedel's thyroiditis.
- Attempt to feel for any discrete thyroid nodule. These are best appreciated using the pulp of your examining fingers (second, third, and fourth digits).
- Ask the patient to swallow during palpation, and check for any retrosternal extension of the thyroid gland.
- Grade thyromegaly with the WHO classification system (see Sect. 2.3.2).
- Palpate all regional lymph node groups (I to VI).

Percussion

- Percussion of the sternal manubrium may be required in patients with a suspected retrosternal goiter. The percussion note will be dull. This step is seldom warranted, especially if there is no palpable thyroid tissue extending below the proximal portion of the manubrium (thoracic aperture).

Auscultation

- In patients with hyperdynamic circulation, as might occur in overt Graves' disease, a bruit may be appreciated over the superior poles of the thyroid in the vicinity of the superior thyroid arteries.

Appendix 3: Mnemonics in Endocrinology

Pheochromocytomas (the 10 Percent Rule)
- 10% are familial
- 10% are malignant
- 10% are extra-adrenal

More recent evidence points to a genetic cause of pheochromocytomas in up to 30% of patients. This mnemonic provides an understanding of the general behavior of these tumors.

Pheochromocytomas (8Ps of Presentation)
- Pallor (*not* flushing)
- Perspiration
- Panic
- Pain (headache)
- Postural dizziness
- Panic attack
- Palpitations
- Paradoxical hypertension in the setting of beta-receptor blockers

Insulinoma (Rule of 10s)
- 10% are malignant
- 10% are multifocal
- 10% are due to multiple endocrine neoplasia type 1
- 10% are ectopic

Insulinomas are usually unifocal and benign.

Causes of Addison's disease (ADDISON)
- **A**utoimmune adrenalitis (primary adrenal insufficiency)
- **D**rugs (inhibitors of steroidogenesis, ketoconazole, mitotane)
- **D**iffuse amyloid deposition (amyloidosis)
- **I**nfectious agents (tuberculosis, human immunodeficiency virus)
- **S**econdary causes (hypopituitarism)
- **O**ther causes (adrenal hemorrhage)
- **N**eoplasia (usually metastases from primary tumors in the lung, breast, stomach, kidney, rectosigmoid colon or melanoma)

Causes of Diabetic Ketoacidosis (6 Is)
- **I**nfection (urinary or respiratory tract infections)
- **I**nsulinopenia (absolute in type 1 diabetes, relative in type 2 diabetes)
- **I**nfarction (silent myocardial infarction)
- **I**njury (significant trauma or stress)
- **I**ndex presentation (newly diagnosed type 1 diabetes)
- **I**ssues of adherence to insulin therapy

Cause of Hypercalcemia (SHIFT in calcium)
- **S**arcoidosis and other granulomatous diseases
- **H**yperparathyroidism, **h**yperthyroidism, **h**ypervitaminosis A and D
- **I**mmobilization (increased bone resorption)
- **F**amilial (familial hypocalciuric hypercalcemia)
- **T**umors, **t**hiazide diuretics, li**t**hium

Clinical features of Cushing's Syndrome (MOON FACIES)
- **M**enstrual disorders
- **O**steopenia or osteoporosis
- **O**besity (central distribution of fat)
- **N**eurosis (depression or psychosis)
- **F**ace (plethora, hirsutism, acne)
- **A**ltered muscle physiology (proximal muscle weakness)
- Supra**c**lavicular and dorso**c**ervical fat pads
- **I**nfection
- **E**levated blood pressure
- **S**kin (easy bruisability)

Causes of hypoglycemia, FEELING Dizzy
- **F**alse hypoglycemia (pseudohypoglycemia not meeting Whipple's criteria)
- **E**xogenous (insulin or insulin secretagogue)
- **E**thanol
- **L**iver failure
- **I**mmune dysfunction (stimulating anti-insulin antibodies)
- **N**eoplastic (insulinoma or sarcomas producing IGF-2)
- **G**landular dysfunction (pituitary insufficiency, adrenal insufficiency)
- **D**rugs (quinolones, pentamidine, beta-blockers, ACE inhibitors)

Multiple Endocrine Neoplasia *Type 1 (PPP)*
- Pituitary adenoma
- Pancreatic adenoma
- Parathyroid adenoma

Multiple Endocrine Neoplasia Type *2A (MPP)*
- Pheochromocytoma
- Medullary thyroid carcinoma
- Parathyroid adenoma

Multiple Endocrine Neoplasia Type 2B (MPM)
- Pheochromocytoma
- Medullary thyroid carcinoma.
- Mucosal neuromas and a marfanoid body habitus

Management of Osteoporosis (ABCDE)
- **A**ctivity (weight-bearing exercise)
- **B**isphosphonates
- **C**alcium supplementation
- **D** (vitamin D supplementation)
- **E**strogens (menopausal hormone therapy)

Causes of Gynecomastia (MAKE BREAST)
- **M**arijuana
- **A**lcohol
- **K**linefelter's syndrome
- **E**strogen excess
- **B**aby (circulating maternal estrogens)
- **R**eceptor blockers (ketoconazole, calcium channel blockers, and H2 blockers)
- **E**lderly
- **A**ntineoplastic agents (alkylating agents)
- **S**pironolactone
- **T**umors (adrenal or testicular)

Index

© Springer Nature Switzerland AG 2020   193
A. Manni, A. Quarde, *Endocrine Pathophysiology*,
https://doi.org/10.1007/978-3-030-49872-6

Printed in the United States
By Bookmasters